PHOOLPROOF

ADVANCE PRAISE FOR *PHOOLPROOF*

'Jhelum calls herself a flower witch. And she is. [S]he takes you through the various aspects of blooms with incantations that cast a spell on you'—Nonita Kalra, editor, *Harper's Bazaar*

'What a fascinating read! Having known Jhelum in my working life as a chronicler of beauty, it is so logical that she should be the author of this amazing journey into the world of beauty, healing and spiritual guidance with flowers. So much to learn and understand . . . Superbly collated and poetically expressed'—Cory Walia, make-up artist

'I was a follower of Bach flower therapy, which somewhere had got lost. I am so glad that Jhelum has brought this beautiful philosophy back into my life with *Phoolproof*. The book is well-researched and opens up many channels of healing with flowers. Kudos to Jhelum for this lovely rediscovery and for gently leading us into the mystical world of Indian blooms—their traditions, legends and the healing power of nature—and its world of happiness'—Nayanika Chatterjee, supermodel

'With my busy schedule, I could only skim through *Phoolproof* but Jhelum's writing caught my attention from the first chapter itself. I love the way she has weaved in her poetry with history, nostalgia and healing, and has offered such simple remedies. I am impressed with the wealth of knowledge she has infused into the pages. Each chapter is insightful and evokes a very flowery, colourful imagery. I never knew flowers had so much to offer us! Jhelum has done immense research and I am sure this book is going to help many . . . I am sure going to keep returning to these pages'—Raima Sen, actor

'With *Phoolproof*, Jhelum Biswas Bose opens a door to a fragrant garden of ideas. It blooms with the secrets, legends, myths and mesmeric powers of Indian flowers. She explores their allure, but also the fascinating possibilities they hold—from healing to adornment, essence to emotion—in perfumes, foods and flavours. By sharing bits and pieces of her personal life, her early and abiding fascination with flowers and how they became an almost karmic influence in her life, Bose meanders through anecdotal, historical and remedial stories to argue that flowers matter. Those who will "use" this book of flowers (beyond reading it) for tips on aromatherapy, homeopathic cures, floral oils and concoctions that soothe and heal, perfumes that spark sensuality, face packs and lip balms that prettify and nourish will also find some interesting reflections on the Indian way of life. Not only in Bengali households, where Bose starts her story, but also in the way India culturally connects with flowers. *Gulab, geinda, mogra, rajnigandha* or champak . . . eat, pray and inhale'—Shefalee Vasudev, author, fashion commentator and editor, The Voice of Fashion

'This book is a classic example of how nothing can stop you from climbing unprecedented heights once you find your calling in life' —Rhythma Kaul, deputy health editor, *Hindustan Times*

'I have known Jhelum since the time she was working as the beauty editor at *Harper's Bazaar*. She is as pretty as a rose and warm as a lotus. Her passion for flowers has led to the birth of this amazing book, which makes you believe in flower therapy. From learning to win over your negative emotions to feeling happy and positive about everything in life—this book is a pathway to happiness. This book also gives you remedies for various physical and emotional problems just by using flowers. I have personally tried some of the interesting home remedies and recipes using flowers and have found them amazing. I wish Jhelum all the very best and look forward to many new innovations especially in her product line, Jhelum Loves' —Dr Jaishree Sharad, dermatologist and author

'I remember meeting Jhelum at a *Harper's Bazaar* event more than a decade ago. She was this young, enthusiastic girl wearing a little dress and sporting a short haircut. Before that, I had interacted with her a couple of times and was very impressed with the way she researched her topic before asking questions. The first thing that charmed me about her was the calm in her face and her beautiful smile. It was a serene, loving, warm smile—a lovely greeting. Jhelum left a lasting impression on my mind; and the next time I met her, I called her "my little Buddha" and that phrase just stuck on to our conversations thereafter. Over the years, I've seen her evolve from a beauty journalist and have been after her life to complete her PhD. That's because I saw she was research-oriented, sincere, very passionate and meticulous in what she did—qualities that make her so good at her chosen field that her work quite naturally becomes useful to a larger audience. Such was my Little Buddha.

'And then she wrote this book and asked me to give her my review of the same. Me being me, I kept putting it off because I had a tight schedule. And at last she sent me a very gentle reminder, and then, "Deadline!" That got me reading the book and I just couldn't put it down.

'*Phoolproof* is a wealth of knowledge. I knew of Bach flower remedy, have a clinical degree in acupuncture and am attuned to Ayurveda . . . I already had an interest in alternative healing. So when I read her book, I could see how authentic Jhelum's research is, how beautifully she has compiled that into the book and infused it with poetry, anecdotes and legends from our rich culture and heritage. She has picked from everything that is authentic and then proved it with modern scientific knowledge. I think this was one of the nicest books I've read on beauty and it reminded me of something my dad had told me: "a doctor needs to have *kayiguna*", which is a Kannada phrase where "kayi" means hand, and "guna", talent . . . The word kayiguna means "blessing in your hand" . . . I feel Jhelum has that quality . . . that healing touch.

'Jhelum, lots of love to you, the book is fantastic! I'm going to keep it and read it again and again'—Dr Rashmi Shetty, dermatologist and author

'*Phoolproof* is a fascinating read about the amazing world of flowers and their magic in our daily lives. My best wishes and luck to Jhelum'—Mimi Chakraborty, actor and parliamentarian

'Jhelum and I met through work when she was the beauty editor of *Harper's Bazaar* and we instantly found a common language—we Bengalis literally smell each other out and address a few words to each other, which can't be translated as they lose their essence—and connected quite naturally. We kept in touch over the years and I observed her every move of building a brand—Jhelum Loves—with much dedication and passion. I absolutely love these products and felt honoured when she created a perfume dedicated to me. It was a pleasure to read her book, *Phoolproof*, which again is a work created with much passion and dedication. It truly makes for a "beauty-phool" read'—Kalyani Saha Chawla, entrepreneur

'Brilliant work, well explained! This book reflects Jhelum's passion for plant and flower remedies'—Dr Ravi Ratan Sharma, perfumer and alternative healer

'I have known Jhelum for over a decade now, when she had just about started her career as a beauty writer with *Good Housekeeping* magazine. We continued working very closely and did some memorable shoots together when she was the beauty editor of *Harper's Bazaar*. Over the years we have become good friends and continue to exchange notes on beauty. Reading her book, *Phoolproof*, has been an absolute delight. It is a beautifully written book, penned with Jhelum's trademark dedication and passion. It is an in-depth work on nature's most amazing creation—flowers! This poetically written book with its stories, remedies, rituals and recipes is a must-read for everyone' —Anu Kaushik, make-up artist

'Jhelum has done a "foolproof" job of making us discover the immense good power of flowers (Indian flowers) on us . . . on our body, on our mind and on our soul. She combined all her passions into this book—her love for words, flowers, healing and yoga. In fact, she has experienced the healing power of flowers on herself—they cured her breathing troubles . . . and breath is the cornerstone of skillful and mindful living. As a fellow yoga practitioner, avid scuba driver and adventure motorcyclist, this book resonates with me at different levels of natural beauty, of healing and self-enhancement'—Dinesh Dayal, President, IBHA (Indian Beauty and Hygiene Association); CEO and Founder, La Terre Growth Advisors; Associate Partner, Helix International Paris

'A sense of serenity is what I always take away from meeting Jhelum. She heals without knowing that she's doing it. Which is why I was overwhelmed when she told me that she had created one of her earlier perfumes, Flambe, with me in mind (she used the word muse, can you believe it?). The first time I used it, I felt like I had worn it all my life. This is the reason I always look to Jhelum for advice on aromas, healing, cooking, relationships and even life. And how different are these all, really? Jhelum truly is, as she mentions in her opening lines, a flower witch. The good kind'—Varun Rana, Content Lead, Good Earth

'I have known Jhelum for a long time and the passion that I have seen in her has been as beautiful as this book. This book is a great initiative to encourage people to understand the usage of flowers in therapeutic ways in today's stressful lives'—Dr Mahima Bakshi, author and wellness consultant

'Jhelum Biswas Bose has approached *Phoolproof* the same way she does everything in her life, with hard work and sincerity. She reaches out to people and nurtures relationships, and the book is built on that foundation. *Phoolproof* touches on various aspects of flowers that I hadn't ever thought about: Mary Magdalene's essential oils, Mehrunisa's love for roses and Madurai *malligai*'s GI tag. There are poems, myths and healing advice, all meant as a gentle reminder that flowers go beyond their ornamental value.

'As a former health journalist, it is easy to bring plants down to what they can give us: antioxidants that have healing properties. Most of us are busy trying to "extract" what we can from nature as we go about our hectic daily life. *Phoolproof* is telling us to slow down—to wind a rose petal around a pod of *elaichi* and chew on it, so the flavour explodes in our mouths. It helps us live with flowers, not exploit them for their beauty and goodness. It's a good book to read if you're looking for solutions other than allopathy to help you deal with anxiety or stress. Mostly, though, it's a book from a person who identifies as a flower witch. Surely, we must pay attention'—Sunalini Mathew, journalist, *The Hindu*

'With *Phoolproof*, Jhelum Biswas Bose opens up the world of flowers and their effect on the human body and psyche. Deeply informative, yet easy to read, the book is brought to life with personal anecdotes, recipes, poems and her years of experience as a beauty editor, [Bach flower remedies] practitioner and creator of Jhelum Loves. It made me want to rush-order floral oils and essences and start creating my own beauty regime'—Nishat Fatima, former editor, *Harper's Bazaar*; author; and photographer

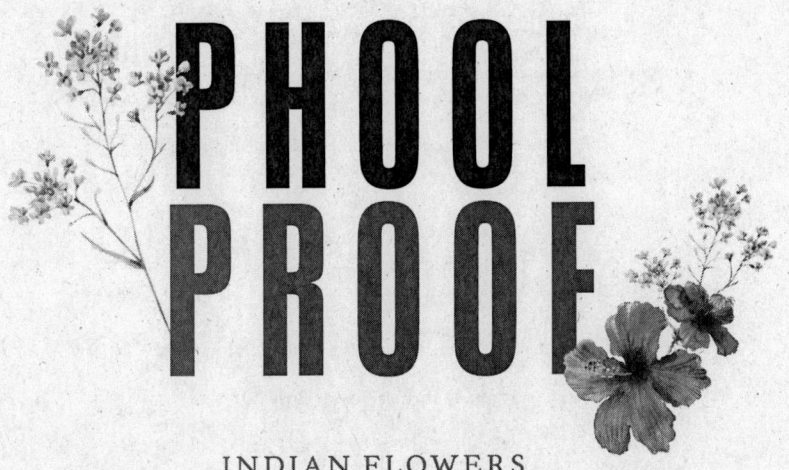

PHOOL PROOF

INDIAN FLOWERS, THEIR MYTHS, TRADITIONS & USAGE

JHELUM BISWAS BOSE

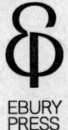

EBURY
PRESS

An imprint of Penguin Random House

EBURY PRESS

USA | Canada | UK | Ireland | Australia
New Zealand | India | South Africa | China | Singapore

Ebury Press is part of the Penguin Random House group of companies
whose addresses can be found at global.penguinrandomhouse.com

Published by Penguin Random House India Pvt. Ltd
4th Floor, Capital Tower 1, MG Road,
Gurugram 122 002, Haryana, India

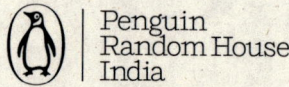

Penguin
Random House
India

First published in Ebury Press by Penguin Random House India 2019

Copyright © Jhelum Biswas Bose 2019

Flower illustrations by Sahitya Rani

ISBN 9780143447221

Typeset in Adobe Garamond Pro by Manipal Digital Systems, Manipal

Printed at Repro India Limited

www.penguin.co.in

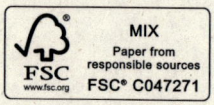

MIX
Paper from
responsible sources
FSC® C047271

To Gotan (Gautam Ghosh, my uncle and guide) and Gunjan (my friend for eternity)—who left me a little too early. While Gotan with his wisdom taught me many a life lesson—the foremost being 'do what you dream'—Gunjan with her passion for love and life always brought the light of cheer into the gloomiest of my days. I miss them both, but I am also convinced that today, wherever they are, they are both cheering me on. Gotan, I know I have your blessings with me every moment. And, my dear Gunjan, I can hear your exuberant laugh in my ears, daring me to take on another flight of fantasy.

May you live in such a way
that others will say,
'She is a woman
who, though ordinary,
somehow stands out
and has a beautiful story to tell.'

—Dr Daisaku Ikeda

CONTENTS

FOREWORD

When Jhelum approached me to write the foreword for *Phoolproof*, I had the opportunity to reacquaint myself with nature, healing and the charm of everyday spells. While the world Jhelum writes about initially seemed unrelated to me, once I took a pause to read, reflect and immerse myself in her story, I was reminded of the old adage—many paths, one goal.

Phoolproof is a paean to flowers and healing that, at the same time, evokes the metaphorical flower that never withers inside you. In India, we are rarely far from flowers—in the form of offerings, decoration or celebration—and are in an enduring relationship with rose water, attar and a spectrum of fragrances. Yet, we may remain oblivious to the pervasive power of scent: to trigger, to transform and to heal.

In modern life, we are all archers walking towards a city of answers, taking aim with the hope that our target will reveal the near-silent stories of our hearts and spirit beneath the surface of the business and busyness of life. There is a living world around us; treasure-like precious healing ingredients, flowers and medicines which release wild mercies and ecstatic gratitude of the spirit: the lost language— if you will—of the natural world. But these are not just spells. These remedies are practical, rooted in enhancing our reality and keeping us mindful and grounded. Jhelum's infectious flower philosophy caught me in its seductive net. I've come to understand through my own healing journey that to devote one's time and effort to the divine can be an act of resistance, but also essential.

I found myself smoothing on oils mixed by Jhelum, closing my eyes and recalling strings of mogra from my childhood; the ripeness of petrichor vibrating in the air on the eve of monsoon; and the enchantment of lotus and aromas, like wish-fulfilling gems, armed with mysterious properties.

This book offers a way of reclaiming the divine in our daily life.

May you be inspired to do the same.

Lisa Ray, author and actor

INTRODUCTION

FINDING MY TRIBE

From a scholar pursuing research in English literature from Jawaharlal Nehru University, New Delhi; landing myself in the fancy job of a beauty editor with *Harper's Bazaar*, India, followed by a brief stint in the retail industry as the marketing head of Sephora India and Satya Paul; to then giving it all up at the peak of my career to start my own beauty website (Beauty Beats) and a social media consultancy (Candied Communication); studying alternative healing philosophies of Bach flower remedy, aromatherapy, yoga and chakra healing to become a certified healer; creating a beauty brand called Jhelum Loves; and writing this book on flower therapy—my career has been diverse and varied.

Hence, when I am asked what I do, I am not sure where to start and what to say. At times I call myself an entrepreneur, sometimes a healer, occasionally a writer, a beauty commentator, a poet and quite often—for a little drama and attention—I say, 'I am a flower witch!' Why do

I call myself a flower witch? Well, because, as I said, I like the instant attention I get when I say that. However, on a serious note, I say that because I do believe I am indeed a flower witch.

Who is a witch?

- Is she someone who stirs up unusual recipes? Then, yes, I do that. I love cooking innovative dishes. I also create healing beauty products with natural ingredients.
- Is a witch someone who speaks to forces of nature in riddles and rhymes? Well, then I do speak to flowers and converse with them through poems and songs.
- Is she someone who doesn't walk the beaten track? One only needs to look at my career graph to know that I have indeed constantly changed gears and traversed diverse paths.
- Does she fly off on a broom? I don't do that, but I do fly off in my dreams and fancies.
- Is she someone who faces opposition for being different? My life has indeed been rife with obstacles and I have often been questioned for my choices.

Therefore, I feel I do qualify to be a witch of sorts. That brings us to the next question: Why 'flower' witch?

WHY FLOWERS?

Since early childhood I have been drawn to the beauty of fresh flowers. From my earliest memories I remember, every morning, fresh *bela* (*Jasminum sambac*) or *juhil jui* (*Jasminum auriculatum*) would be picked from our terrace garden and offered to the pantheon of gods in our prayer room. On Saturdays, red hibiscus (or what is popularly known as *jaba* in Bengali) and *aprajita* (blue peony) would be offered to Ma Kali and Shiva; on Thursdays, the neighbourhood *phoolwala* would get *kamal* (lotus) for Lakshmi puja and, on Durga puja, 108 pink kamals would be offered at the pandal.

My mother would always keep our living room daintily decorated with fresh flowers and her handmade ribbon flowers. During our holidays, I would observe her picking up wild flowers and tucking a bloom behind her ear. Her love for flowers inspired her to often dress me up as a Kashmiri flower girl for fancy-dress parties or contests. I guess my name, and my own developing love for flowers, helped do justice to her passion.

My grandmothers—paternal (Thakuma) and maternal (Didu) both—were also very fond of flowers. While Thakuma would love to keep a bowl of bela flowers in her room, Didu preferred the golden champak. It's not surprising that both had named their daughters after flowers. My *pishi* (father's sister) is called Jui and my *maashi* (mother's sister) is called Jaba. As I grew up, I was fascinated by floral essential oils and fragrances, and soon enough, and very naturally, flowers became an integral part of my life.

I never used deodorants; I would use essential oils instead. During summer breaks I learnt ribbon flower–making and ikebana; and in winters I learnt how to tend to a garden. However, as I grew up and got entangled in life's challenges and complications, somewhere I lost touch with flowers.

THE STORY OF MY LIFE

From early childhood I was prone to cold and cough. However, this condition worsened as I grew older. For years I lived on antibiotics and didn't know what it felt like to breathe easy. It took a huge toll on my quality of life while I was working at Satya Paul. Things took such a dark turn that I had no choice but to take a sabbatical from work. I had already exhausted all possible allopathic treatments, and that's when an acquaintance advised me to start yoga therapy. Practising yoga helped me to slowly heal my body and mind, and encouraged me to explore alternative healing therapies.

Practising Nichiren Daishonin's Buddhism, I treated this challenge as an opportunity to transform my life. I took the sabbatical to ponder on what I wished to do with my life. My mother, Ruby Biswas, who is a renowned make-up artist and aesthetician in Calcutta, had always wanted me to do a course in make-up. Now that I had the time, I enrolled for a course in make-up in University of Arts, London. There, during a weekend I did a weekend course on Bach flower remedies from Ainsworths. This fascinated me and, thereafter, I completed all three levels of Bach flower remedy, and am now a recognized Bach foundation registered practitioner (BFRP) and practise this therapy to heal people by helping them heal their emotions.

Post that, I trained to become an aromatherapist, chakra healer and yoga expert. Combining these healing therapies, what I have developed is a comprehensive practice that I refer to as flower therapy. Through this practice I have been able to heal and help many others.

RETURN OF THE FLOWERS

With these therapies, flowers have quite naturally re-entered my life. Now, in my home, flowers bloom in the tiny balconies; fresh flowers liven up my living spaces; floral prints and embroidery fill my wardrobe; and hairpins with flowers have found their way to style my hair; and lately they occupy also my kitchen and beauty cabinet. My connection with flowers has deepened my understanding of myself and connected me to nature. Over the years I have learnt to recognize and respect the subtle energies of blooms.

If you feel a similar affinity towards flowers, then rest assured: You have found a kindred spirit and are holding a book that speaks your language.

HOW TO READ THIS BOOK?

NAVIGATING THE PAGES

Ideally, I would say read this book in its chronological order. However, I feel you can dip in anywhere to understand the language and power of flowers. The book has been structured in five parts:

LORES & LEGENDS: This section gives you a peek into the mystical world of flowers and the myths associated with these gorgeous blooms.

ESSENCE & EMOTIONS: In this section you will gain a basic understanding of different flower essences and how they can heal your emotions. It also guides you on how to make your own flower remedies.

SCENT & SENSUALITY: Here, I have shared my knowledge of essential oils and how to incorporate them in your life to heal your skin, hair and mind, and make natural, healing perfume blends.

ADORNMENTS & ANOINTMENTS: This section includes numerous recipes for using flowers in personal grooming.

FOODS & FLAVOURS: This section is a collection of recipes for using flowers in your daily meals.

PART I

LORES & LEGENDS

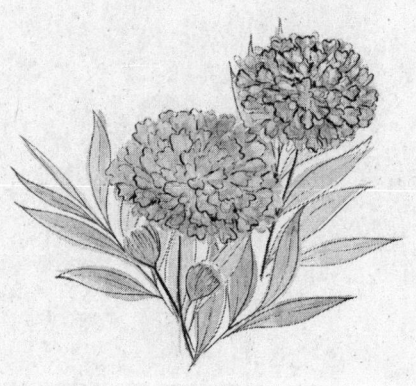

TELLING TALES

If you are a Bengali girl born and brought up in Calcutta, you will have surely learnt either singing and/or dancing. And the first song and dance that you would have learnt is invariably '*Phoole phoole dhole dhole*' by Rabindranath Tagore. I loved this dreamy, easy song, and enjoyed swaying like a flower to its lilting tunes. As is with most Indian households, whenever guests are over, the child in the house is asked to sing a song, dance or recite a poem, basically just do something to entertain the guests and make parents proud that indeed their child is learning something in their extra-curricular classes. While most children shy away or find it embarrassing, I would never miss an opportunity to sing and dance to '*Phoole phoole dhole dhole*', even though I was timid and introverted.

Today, when I analyse what made me so excited about that song and dance, I feel a lot had to do with the fact that I loved flowers, and that every time I performed it on stage I would get to wear bela garlands in my hair and a saree.

FLOWERS IN FAIRY TALES

Listening to and reading fairy tales was something I loved since early childhood. The first book I remember reading was a large, thin book that told the tale of 'Thumbelina'—a tiny girl who emerged from a barley flower and was as high as a thumb. I loved Thumbelina's walnut-shell bed, rose-petal cover and the lotus leaf that protected her. Thumbelina's adventures and her victory taught me very early in life that no matter how small or insignificant you may think you are you have the power to win over every adversity, provided you are determined to do so.

In one book, I came across beautiful illustrations of the story. They led me to dream up a complete film reel on Thumbelina and her adventures.

I would bend into flowers to see if there were tiny people living within them. Sometimes, I would think I saw them . . . Not exactly saw . . . but, you know, just a movement, a little spark, a bit of pollen dust, a pair of tiny wings fluttering—could have been butterflies . . .

Okay, I admit I believed and I still do believe in flowers and fairies. When you let your imagination flow, this world opens its doors to you. It is such a beautiful feeling that there are subtle energies around you, playing with you, making you smile and protecting you. The more I surround myself with flowers, the more my intuition sharpens and my sensitivities deepen.

Apart from 'Thumbelina', there are various other fairy tales that have flowers as characters or as important props/symbols. In 'Red Riding Hood', the wolf leads the little girl astray by convincing her to pick flowers for her grandmother. In 'Snow White and Red Rose', the rose creepers play a significant role. In 'Rapunzel', the witch's flower garden is a crucial aspect of the story. Flowers also abound in Indian fairy tales like '*Lal Kamal aur Neel Kamal*', '*Shaath Bhai Champa*' and 'King Paari and the Jasmine Creeper'.

FLORAL LEGENDS

Flowers are not just elements of folklore; they are legends in themselves. While I have shared several myths and tales on flowers in later pages, here are some of my favourites. I particularly like the story of *parijaat* flowers, also known as *shiuli* or *harshingar*. The poem below is my retelling of the story:

'Parijaat Was Her Name'

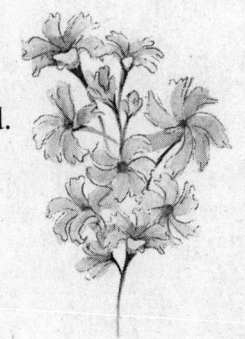

Her delicate skin
turned crimson when the sun kissed.
Yet her deep dark eyes
trailed the sun god
as he traversed
from East to West.

He scorched her skin,
yet she was ready to burn,
as long as every nightfall he returned.

Surya, the sun god, knew her heart,
that to be with him, her delicate form
would move heaven and earth.
So in the bitter winter,
he came down to her palace door,
and suddenly it was like spring.
Butterflies flapped their wings,
bees hummed, squirrels played;
the birds sang and flowers bloomed.

For a while Nature thought
spring would forever be.
But come February,
the weather got hot and sultry.

We would call it global warming,
but in those times
the heavenly deities
didn't fear these calamities.

Surya realized
that for lives to survive
love has to be sacrificed,
and he must return to the skies.

Resigned to his fate,
Surya set out towards the sky.
But seeing him soar,
Princess Parijaat desperately clung on,
to a ray of hope.

She raced to the heavens
and was soon burnt to ashes.

The gods and goddesses cried,
tears of grief and sorrow
fell on the fragrant ashes,
like beautiful heavenly shower.
And from the remains of that lover,
a passionate tree emerged.

Shiuli was its name.
Its white flowers bloom in October
and hold a ray of sunshine
in its heart centre.

It's believed that in the autumn night,
Surya visits his beloved,
but at dawn returns to his heavenly abode,
that as he kisses her goodbye,
she heaves a sigh.

That the night blooms let out a fragrant breath,
and the ground beneath
looks like a nuptial bed.

Another romantic Indian tale I find very poetic and sensual is the story of Kamadeva and his five floral arrows. Ayurvedic specialist Dr Ipsita Chatterjee from Delhi, who has extensively helped me with her expertise in Ayurveda, shared this fascinating legend with me. According to ancient folklore, Kamadeva, the Indian version of Cupid, carries five arrows with which he pierces the senses of his victims. His bow is made of sugarcane and the bowstring is coated with honey. The five types of arrows have five different arrowheads. They are: *aravinda* (white lotus), *ashoka* (sorrow-less tree), *cuta* (mango flower), *navamallika* (jasmine) and *nilotpala* (blue lotus). These five floral arrows also represent five kinds of desire—*unmada*, *tapana*, *shudhana*, *stambhana* and *sammohana* respectively.

If this fascinates you, then I recommend you read the book *Five Arrows of Kama*: *The Art of Love, Sex and Desire* by Sandhya Mulchandani. It is a collection of translations of five erotic texts from medieval India: *Pururavasa Manasijasutram*, *Narmakelikutuhala Samvadam*, *Smarapradipika*, *Manmatha Samhita* and *Kadambari Swikaranakarika*.

NATURE POETRY

Flowers have often inspired poetry, especially Romantic poetry. Who can forget William Wordsworth's 'I Wandered Lonely as a Cloud', where the poet shares how his sadness dissolves the moment he sees 'a host . . . of golden daffodils'. Or for that matter, John Keats's 'Ode to Autumn', where the reaper falls asleep in the fields: 'Drowsed with the fume of poppies, while thy hook/Spares the next swath and all its twined flowers . . .'

Closer home, Rabindranath Tagore's songs and poems on seasons are ingrained in every Bengali's psyche. In today's world, one may hardly ever experience the nuances of the six Indian seasons like Tagore's popular songs might help one imagine. '*Esho hey boishak*' welcomed summer; '*Khoro bayu boy bege*' celebrated the monsoon winds; '*Megher kole rod hesheche*' bid adieu to the monsoons, and welcomed the sunny days of early autumn ('Hey Hemantalakshmi', where the season of *hemanta* [late autumn] is viewed as Goddess Lakshmi).

However, much before Keats or Tagore eulogized the seasons, there was Kalidasa, the great poet of medieval India, who waxed eloquent on nature and its beauty in his collection of poems *Ritusamharam* (literally: 'garland of seasons'). The text is divided into six sections, celebrating the beauty of nature in the six seasons and how lovers respond to each of them. It's amorous, raw, sensuous and passionate. And what I like the best about these verses is the seductive use of flowers to describe the sensations of the season.

FLOWERS & THE FEMININE

Traditionally, in almost every culture, flowers were used to describe feminine beauty and praise the physical beauty of women. Perhaps it was quite a logical thing to do. After all, flowers contain the reproductive organs of a plant. It's commonplace to equate flower buds to virginity and flowers in general to purity. And possibly to sanctify the purity even further, flowers are often used to depict the beauty of goddesses. For instance, Goddess Gauri, an incarnation of Parvati, is described to have feet as shapely and dainty as lotus petals.

In Christianity, a biblical passage from the Song of Solomon—'I am a rose of Sharon, a lily of the valley'—has often been interpreted as a reference to the Virgin Mary. Hence, it's no surprise that representations of Mother Mary often include lily as a symbol of purity and virginity—or rose as a mark of love and beauty.

Once associated with divinity, flowers easily became symbols of purity and, therefore, quite naturally, started getting used to depict female beauty and virtue. Kalidasa in *Ritusamharam* describes a woman's glowing complexion to a freshly bloomed lotus and her twinkling eyes to blue lilies.

In his most famous work, *Abhijnana Shakuntalam*, when Shakuntala firsts appears on stage, her friend describes her to be as dainty as a jasmine. Shakuntala says that she tends to flowers the way she would tend to her sisters. Shakuntala's youthful body is compared to that of a young blooming flower, her delicate form to the petals of blue lotus, and her lips are described as red blooms.

FLOWERS OF HOPE

Flowers have been compared to all things beautiful, through all ages. I don't think any civilization ever has seen flowers as being ugly or inauspicious. However, for me, the most touching symbolism of a flower bloom is its depiction as a source of hope. In August 2018, when floods ravaged Kerala, optimism was reinforced in people's hearts when *neelakurinji* flowers blossomed gregariously in the hills of Munnar immediately after the floods. It was a rare sight, as the kurinji blooms only once in twelve years. One can only imagine what joy this would have brought to those who suffered this natural disaster.

My balcony and the trees around my house have also taught me some valuable lessons in life. I remember walking home one exceptionally warm November evening, when I was upset about something (I can't even remember what). And then, suddenly, a sweet, heady aroma filled my breath and I felt soft, tiny white blossoms on my head. This kind gesture from nature instantly changed my mood and made me realize that life has to be lived in each moment.

PART 2

ESSENCE & EMOTIONS

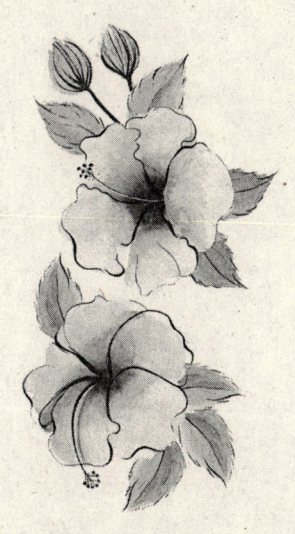

DISCOVERING BACH FLOWER REMEDIES

This book wouldn't have happened, and my life would have not taken the turn that it did, had it not been for Bach flower remedies.

'Flowers, My Friends'

Since early childhood I have been fragile.
So much so that I could swoon
(I was told),
even if it were just a flower that was at me thrown.
Now why would you throw a flower?
I would wonder . . .
Aren't blooms beautiful enough to be treasured?
Did you not see the fairies handle them with so much care?
'You are reading so much of Grimm's Fairy Tales,'
I was told.
'They are filling your mind with silly imagination.'
But . . . but did you really not see those wings flutter?
Did you not see them,
lying on the bed of shiuli,
in the early morning hours of October?
Did you not see them seated atop a bee,
and enter the honeysuckle flower's territory?

On one summer break,
I made crowns, garlands and bracelets,
of jasmine and *champa* flowers.
I wore them and walked about,
telling anyone who cared to lend an ear . . .
All that glitters is not gold.
See here, in these blooms you will find
golden-yellow fairy dust,
and a small shot of flower juice.
One day I heard my mother say,
Cleopatra bathed in milk and rose.
She may have been a queen,
but why should I be any less?
I thought.
So in a tub of water,
I poured in milk powder,
and put in some petals of red rose.
I spent a couple of hours bathing like a queen,
and came out with a blocked nose,
and clogged drains in the shower.
That night and two nights after,
my body burned with raging fever.
Pneumonia, the doctor declared;
no more flowers, fairies and rain.
Antibiotics, antihistamines
were to be my support from hence.
Cold and cough became my
eternal opponents.
Friends drew caricatures
of me and my running nose.

Limericks were written
on my perennial woes.
Here I quote, from what one of the many a friend wrote:
'There was once a maiden by the name of a river.
Coughs and colds would give her a shiver.
Her nose would always be as red as rose,
Two Cetirizines were her daily dose.
That sneezing maiden by the name of a river.'

Years passed,
battles raged.
Stress, worries and lifestyle
further damaged my condition.
I felt my body
had prematurely aged.
I gasped for breath,
coughed and sneezed,
till to my bones I ached.
The doctors said,
avoid pollution and stress.

I replied,
I can move to the Himalayas for fresh air,
but who says there'll be no stress there?
This continued till 2010,
when flowers returned to my life again.
A family friend—a fairy godmother of sorts—
introduced me to Bach flower remedies.
Her magic potion,
in a little amber bottle,

worked nothing short of a miracle.
My worries eased,
with that my sneezing ceased.
Slowly I gained confidence in myself,
and I don't know when
cold and cough disappeared.
The essence healed me,
and intrigued me;
I wanted to know more . . .

The family friend who introduced me to Bach flower remedies, Neeta Sabharwal, explained that these were a mix of flower essences—Rescue Remedy and crab apple—and advised me to always keep them handy at home. From then on, each time I would have a complaint, she would have a remedy! Olive for when I felt unusually tired, scleranthus for my vertigo, honeysuckle to tide over the moments when I mourned my grandmother. I had no idea, though, why these medicines were given for the said situations. I simply took them with water (four drops, four times a day) because they made me feel exponentially better. It eventually also dawned on me that many months had passed by without me having to take any antibiotics. I decided that I wanted to know more about these remedies. I started diligently researching and, over the years, completed three levels of a practitioner's course. I, now, use these remedies to heal myself, my family and friends, and clients.

WHAT ARE BACH FLOWER REMEDIES?

Bach flower remedies are thirty-eight flower essences that comprise a complete system of alternative healing. These flower remedies were discovered by Dr Edward Bach in the 1930s in England. Dr Bach was a physician and homeopath. He believed that attitude, mind and emotions played a vital role in the health and well-being of an individual, and when a person's emotions were 'balanced' or restored to their positive potential, the health improved and ailments could in turn be cured.

The principle of flower essences is similar to any other vibrational healing therapy. Flowers have unique energies, and when the 'essences' of these flowers are taken by us, they affect our vibrations and bring in a balance. They are chosen based on the current emotions or personality of the individual. Therefore, you will not be given a remedy for your headache but for your emotional state while experiencing the headache. For instance, if I am having a headache I may get extremely irritable and impatient and, therefore, I may have to take impatiens Bach flower remedy, while another person when experiencing the headache may suffer silently because she doesn't want to bother others. Such a person may require agrimony. Yet another individual can get so perturbed by it that she will continue talking about it and disturb others. She would require heather or chicory Bach flower remedies.

TRADITION OF FLOWER REMEDIES

Though Bach flower remedies are fast gaining popularity, they are neither 'new' nor the only type of flower essences that mankind has seen. The therapeutic use of flower essences dates back some 10,000 years to the aborigines of Australia. It is believed that this ancient tribe not only used flower essences in their ceremonial practices but also in healing 'flower saunas'—a tradition in which they dug up a pit, filled it with wild flowers and then immersed a person into it to heal him or her. This practice is continued till date in the country. A Buddhist tradition of flower essence therapy in Malaysia and Thailand, where temples specialize in flower-essence healing, is also still in practice. Ayurveda, and Chinese and Tibetan medicinal systems— in fact, most indigenous cultures across the world—have used and continue to use flower waters for healing in some form or other. Since the 1980s, there has been a fresh and renewed interest in flower essences across the globe. The Bush Flower Essences of Australia developed by Ian White, Desert Alchemy of Arizona by Cynthia Athina Kemp (now Kemp-Scherer), Aloha Flower Essences of Hawaii by Penny Medeiros, New Perception Flower Essences of New Zealand by (the now late) Mary Garbely, and Flower Cure of India by the late Dr Malti Khaitan are some of the schools of flower remedy that developed in the late twentieth century. Most of them were in some way or the other influenced by Dr Bach's scholarship, and their endeavour has been to localize and, at the same time, expand the possibilities of flower water healing. However, the system of flower essences I feel is the most comprehensive, effective, adaptable and is more easily available is the Bach flower remedies.

FLOWER ESSENCES AND ESSENTIAL OILS

People often assume that flower essences are floral essential oils or aromatic oils that are extracted from flowers. They are complex compounds like terpenes, esters, aldehydes, ketones, alcohols, phenols and oxides, which make them highly therapeutic. More details about essential oils are covered in the next section, Scents & Sensuality.

Flower essences are flower infusions/concoctions/ tinctures that are consumed for healing the mind, body and soul. It is believed that flowers hold the essence or the life force of the plant, and when water is infused with flowers, the imprint of that particular floral energy is taken up by the water crystals and then preserved when diluted with high-grade alcohol. Hence, when we consume this 'energized' water, the flower energy finds a resonance with the vibrations of our body. This action creates a balance of energies within us and, thereby balances our emotions.

WHERE CAN ONE SOURCE BACH FLOWERS FROM?

Bach flower remedy users or practitioners don't really source the flowers. What we use are bottled remedies, which are available from different homeopathy brands in India, or are bought from stores like Nelsons and Boots when travelling abroad. While purists of the tradition advocate getting the 'original' remedies—essences that are made by Nelsons according to Dr Bach's original method at The Bach Centre in UK—in my experience, remedies from Indian companies work equally well and are definitely far easier to access. I have my personal kit of the 'original' remedies, but I extensively use the ones from the popular Indian, Delhi-based homeopathy brand Bhandari Homeopathy.

BACH FLOWER THERAPY AND HOMEOPATHY

Dr Bach's method of preparing mother tinctures of his flower remedies appears to be similar to the methods of homeopathy tincture. And though the Bach flower remedies are available in India in select homeopathy stores, manufactured by leading homeopathy companies in the country, and recommended by some homeopathy physicians, these remedies are not a part or subgroup of homeopathy.

DO THE REMEDIES REALLY WORK?

That's a very legitimate question and it should cross your mind. The answer to it is: Yes, these remedies can heal us. However, a lot of the healing involves a self-transformation in your emotional state. When you go for a Bach flower consultation, you are gently led to recognize your own emotions. Just the process of recognizing your feelings can be extremely healing.

For instance, I suffered from chronic cold, and any slight change in temperature, climate or personal/professional life would trigger it. I started taking walnut Bach flower remedy, a flower essence that helps us accept change. I also took crab apple Bach flower remedy with it to get rid of negativity. Together, these remedies helped me clear my mind and accept change as the single-most important fact of life. As my attitude changed, slowly my chronic ailment disappeared.

Dr Bach believed that these remedies in different combinations can balance and heal any emotions. It is important to bear in mind that the remedies won't suppress negative emotions; rather they will raise your vibrations or improve your life state to develop positive emotions, the way, for instance, music works in uplifting our mood. In other words, the remedies help us understand our troubles and, thereby, empower us to heal ourselves. While acute, extreme emotions get addressed quickly, chronic or prolonged feelings take a while to balance. However, within two weeks, one should be able to perceive a change.

TAKING THE REMEDIES

There are various ways in which you can take the remedies. For beginners, I would recommend the 'glass of water' method, wherein you put two drops of each of your 6–7 chosen remedies—if using Rescue Remedy, take four drops—in a glass of water and sip it through the day. This is best suited for short-term issues.

For chronic problems, it's best to make a remedy mix that will last you 2–3 weeks. In a 30 ml glass bottle with a dropper (you will find it in homeopathy stores, or you can even purchase it online), add two drops of your chosen remedies and/or four drops of Rescue Remedy—if it's a part of your remedy selection—and top it up with mineral water.

From this bottle take four drops directly, or as a mixture with water or a beverage, four times a day. You can also take the remedies 'neat' on your tongue directly. The math is two drops of each chosen remedy and/or four drops of Rescue Remedy. I prefer this method when I am in an emergency situation and need only Rescue Remedy.

I also follow this method when I need short-term remedies like mustard, olive, aspen, elm or cherry plum to address the respective situations: sudden onset of sadness, physical exhaustion, unknown fear, overwhelming work pressure or fear of losing my temper.

THE SIDE EFFECTS

The Bach Centre explains that there are no side effects. In rare cases there may be an upheaval of some negative emotions, but like any other alternative remedy, it is akin to a cleansing effect. If the condition is acute, as in an emergency, take Rescue Remedy till the emotions settle down. Any other symptom is usually coincidental.

WHAT IF I DON'T RESPOND TO THE REMEDIES?

If after about ten days you see no difference at all, ask yourself if you are taking the correct remedies and if you have been taking them correctly. The remedies work very gently and subtly, and at times you may miss out on their nuances. It is, therefore, a good idea to keep a journal to note down your emotions each day. This will help you realize the change when you look back at it after a fortnight or so. Sometimes you may have observed no noticeable change in yourself, but people around may perceive it. Be aware of your own responses and those of others towards you. Being mindful always helps us appreciate subtle energy changes better, which, in turn, work better in our lives.

HOW LONG DO I HAVE TO KEEP TAKING THE REMEDIES?

Our difficulties can be seen as the whorls of an onion. Bach flower remedies help peel away the surface emotions and then the next layer emerges. There's no need to jump the gun and try to unearth what's not apparent. Don't push yourself. Address only what you are prepared to face. Allow the remedies to work and a new layer of emotions emerge. Change your remedies when that happens. This may seem like a continuous process, but then self-improvement is a lifelong process. Bear in mind that the remedies are not habit-forming. Benefits are long-lasting, so you may not have to return to a remedy for a while. However, there may be a relapse, but if you are attuned to the remedies, you will be able to respond quicker.

THE THIRTY-EIGHT REMEDIES

The thirty-eight remedies that are included in Dr Bach's system of flower remedies are listed below with the traits and emotions that they heal:

Agrimony—mental torture behind a cheerful face
Aspen—fear of unknown things
Beech—intolerance
Centaury—the inability to say no
Cerato—lack of trust in one's own decisions
Cherry plum—fear of the mind giving way
Chestnut bud—failure to learn from mistakes

Chicory—selfishness, possessive love

Clematis—dreaming of the future without working in the present

Crab apple—the cleansing remedy, also for self-hatred

Elm—overwhelming feeling of responsibility

Gentian—lack of inspiration caused by a setback

Gorse—hopelessness and despair

Heather—self-centredness and self-concern

Holly—hatred, envy and jealousy

Honeysuckle—living in the past

Hornbeam—tardiness and lethargy

Impatiens—impatience

Larch—lack of confidence

Mimulus—fear of known things

Mustard—deep gloom for no reason

Oak—compulsive plodding beyond the point of exhaustion

Olive—exhaustion following mental or physical effort

Pine—guilt

Red chestnut—over-concern for the welfare of loved ones

Rock rose—terror and fright

Rock water—self-denial, rigidity and self-repression

Scleranthus—inability to choose between alternatives

Star of Bethlehem—shock

Sweet chestnut—extreme mental anguish, when everything has been tried and there is no light left

Vervain—overenthusiasm

Vine—dominance and inflexibility

Walnut—protection from change and unwanted influences

Water violet—quiet self-reliance leading to isolation

White chestnut—unwanted thoughts and mental arguments

Wild oat—uncertainty over one's direction in life
Wild rose—drifting, resignation, apathy
Willow—self-pity and resentment

Rescue Remedy, a mix of five flower remedies—cherry plum, impatiens, star of Bethlehem, clematis and rock rose—to tide over crises or emergencies

CHOOSE YOUR REMEDY

The list above offers a brief overview of the remedies. To start with, you can first think what kind of personality you have and what you are feeling right now, and then check which situations/emotions from the list apply to your current state. Initially, you may feel that you need all or several of them. Go over the list again and make note of the ones that seem to apply to you.

If you are focused enough, your list wouldn't go beyond 10–12 remedies. Now, ponder over this narrowed list and bring it further down to 6–7 remedies. This mix will, in all probability, be the best combination for you.

Another way of familiarizing oneself with the remedies is by starting with Rescue Remedy, when you are in a crisis situation: for example, an accident, an important meeting coming up, or fever. If your strong desire is to get rid of something negative, physical or emotional, then try crab apple.

Incidentally, a combination of Rescue Remedy is excellent for skincare. Mix four drops of each remedy in your face cream or oil or mist to see the difference.

I had a keloid on my right ear for several years. When I began using the remedies, I started applying a few drops of crab apple remedy directly on the keloid and, after about a month, I realized it had reduced to a point where it was noticeable only when attention was drawn to it.

Fatigue is a common experience. If you are feeling physically exhausted after a tiring day, or after recovering from a bout of illness, or if you just feel the need for a caffeine shot, try olive Bach flower remedy. This gentle flower essence has an immediate refreshing effect. However, consulting a Bach flower remedy practitioner is the best bet. You can look up the official Bach Centre webpage, www.bachcentre.com, to find an Indian Bach flower remedy practitioner closest to you.

WHAT'S THE REMEDY FOR STRESS?

That's a question I suppose we all have. But alas! There's no *a* remedy for stress. It wouldn't be appropriate to suggest a remedy for 'stress', because each individual could be stressed for various reasons, and their way of handling stress would be very different. In fact, each individual's cause for stress and level of stress would be different. Further, some people can get stressed for seemingly good things. For instance, one may get stressed with the workload after getting a promotion. Therefore, to correctly address 'stress', it's important to figure out what exactly is the cause of stress. Hence, the person who is getting stressed with a new workload could be given elm to deal with the situation, whereas someone who has been plodding on with many responsibilities for a considerable amount of time may be in need of oak. Yet, someone who is stressed because of the sheer physical exhaustion would require olive.

However, if it's a crisis—like someone has an extremely important decision to make, or there is a sudden crisis at work, or there's been an accident or an urgent need for surgery—then Rescue Remedy can be taken, though I strongly recommend a consultation with a Bach flower remedy practitioner before taking any remedy.

BACH FLOWER REMEDIES AND *CHAKRAS*

Incidentally, Dr Bach had classified the remedies into seven groups based on certain categories of emotions or character traits; and interestingly, he had colour-coded each group. These seven colours happen to be the colours of the rainbow—red, orange, yellow, green, blue, indigo and violet—and hues that are traditionally associated with our seven major chakras (primary energy vortices that we have which control not just our physical systems but also balance our emotions).

While The Bach Centre doesn't really emphasize much on the colour coding, there are some independent Bach flower practitioners (not associated with The Bach Centre in Mount Vernon), like Anna Jeoffroy and Phillip Salmon, who feel there is a deeper significance to the colour coding. Jeoffroy and Salmon opine that perhaps Dr Bach was influenced by the Indian chakra system and thus colour-coded his flower groups based on the colour frequencies associated with the chakras. They feel that the colours that Dr Bach used for each group resonates with the particular chakra that is associated with that group of emotions.

I find this viewpoint very interesting. Incidentally, before completing my three levels of Bach flower therapy from The Bach Centre, I had done a course on Bach flowers from Ainsworths, London, and my teacher for that course was Jeoffroy. Influenced by her reasoning, I do use Bach flower remedies when I am healing chakras, because chakras are connected with emotions.

So yes, if you balance emotions, chakras will also get balanced. For instance, if you are prone to bouts of anger, it is an indication that your solar plexus chakra is imbalanced and you may have issues with digestion. In such a scenario, I would consider holly and/or impatiens to calm your impatience, or dissolve your anger/jealousy, and, thereby, balance the solar plexus chakra.

Hence, my chakra oil blends have remedies that resonate with those chakras. For instance, the first chakra, or the root chakra, is associated with grounding. Therefore, in the chakra oil blend of this chakra, I add the Bach flower remedy of clematis, which helps in bringing the person back to the present, rooting the individual. However, when I am doing a personal consultation and/or personalizing wellness products for a particular individual, while choosing the remedies, I go by the methods that are practised by The Bach Centre, as that keeps the focus clearly on the emotions and the personality. I will share more on chakra healing and my selection of Bach flower remedies later in the section Anointments & Adornments.

THE SEVEN GROUPS

Whether Dr Bach intended these groups to be associated with chakras or not is debatable. However, what it does help in definitely is in understanding the nuances of the remedies and making selection of remedies easier. Given below are the groups and the remedies included in them:

Face Your Fears: mimulus, aspen, rock rose, cherry plum and red chestnut
Live the Day: honeysuckle, clematis, chestnut bud, white chestnut, wild rose, mustard and olive
Reach Out to Others: heather, impatiens, water violet
Know Your Mind: hornbeam, gentian, gorse, scleranthus, wild oat, cerato
Find Joy and Hope: star of Bethlehem, willow, elm, pine, sweet chestnut, larch, oak and crab apple
Live and Let Live: vine, vervain, beech, chicory and rock water
Stand Your Ground: centaury, walnut, holly and agrimony

REMEDIES AND ME

The best thing I like about Bach flower remedies is the fact that each flower essence is like a character. In fact, Dr Bach has written a few short stories on these remedies in a book called *The Story of the Travellers and Other Remedy Stories*. These limericks help me remember the remedies and understand them better. You can also devise associations with these remedies and make your own rhymes, stories or songs around them.

The Bach flower remedies have not just inspired my poetic abilities but have been instrumental in helping me create Jhelum Loves Bach Flower & Aroma Remedies. Most of us know that our health and emotions are reflected in our skin and hair. Through my training in beauty therapy, I was also trained to recognize the emotional trigger that was causing skin/hair issues, but I had no way of addressing their emotional causes. Bach flower remedies helped me bridge that gap, and I realized I could address emotions and thereby treat people inside out.

However, one of the challenges I faced was convincing people to ingest the remedies, as most of them had never heard of this philosophy and doubted its authenticity. In such situations I felt mixing remedies in their beauty products helped. People were open to topical application and, once that showed results, they were ready to take the remedies internally.

For instance, a friend of mine who was prone to acne, as well as sudden and violent bursts of anger, resisted taking cherry plum Bach flower remedy. However, when I mixed it in a bottle of rose water and asked her to spray it on her acne, she agreed readily. Within a week, her skin eruptions subdued and slowly she was able to identify triggers that caused her emotional outbursts. After a month she had glowing skin and was calmer and more self-aware. This dramatic change in her gave me much joy and confidence in my methods.

Meanwhile I had started noticing the difference when I added Bach flower remedies to my own skincare products.

I increasingly started feeling the need for simple products. With my knowledge of aromatherapy, I developed three products—a facewash, a face mist and a face oil. So when people approached me for skin consultations, I spoke to them about Bach flower remedies and, based on my understanding of their situation, I started adding the flower remedies. This helped me personalize each product for each client, and it also helped me understand them better.

In Nichiren Daishonin's Buddhism, which I follow, dialogue and life-to-life interaction are extremely important. The philosophy has helped me become more empathetic and a good listener. It has helped me hear my clients' stories without judgement. In the years 2015–2016, I used Bach flower remedies on a daily basis and, in November 2016, I felt confident enough to do the Level 3 of Bach flower remedies. This four-day workshop helped me hone my skills as a practitioner and clarified the protocol I must follow as a practitioner.

Since then I have been treating Bach flower remedy as a complete system of healing. When clients come for me for a skincare or a haircare consultation, I suggest they, for holistic healing, consult me separately for Bach flower remedies. These separate sessions have enabled me to get a much better understanding of the client. It has also helped them build their faith in me. I have realized that to treat a person I don't need to know every detail of their life. There's no need to prod and goad a person to open up. What is important is to make the person in front feel comfortable and confident enough to share as much as he/she wants to. This approach enables the client to understand himself/herself better and feel in control.

In consciously trying not to push the client I have also learnt not to push myself to own emotions that I am not prepared to accept as yet. In being gentle with myself I have been able to understand and treat myself much better.

I have dealt with my childhood traumas and depression. I am prone to extreme bouts of anger and emotional outbursts. I also go through sudden episodes of anxiety and deep sadness, which sometimes take me to the point of paralysis. In November 2016 I decided to address these concerns with complete focus. I first wanted to deal with my angry outbursts. I realized that in those moments, one of my prominent emotions was the fear of losing control over myself. After discussing this with a fellow practitioner, I started taking cherry plum regularly. Over a month, I recognized the triggers that led me to tip over and, from that realization, I was able to control my outbursts better. Their frequency reduced and so did its intensity. In February 2017, I took cherry plum for only ten days prior to my periods, as that was the time I was more prone to such outbursts, and in March I didn't take it at all.

For my sudden bouts of depression and anxiety, I took mustard and aspen. I kept these remedies close at hand and took them whenever I sensed the cloud of gloom descending over me. Sometimes it gave me instant relief and, at times, I might have to take it for a day.

After taking these remedies I realized that when I am anxious or depressed I usually have one thought or fear stuck in my head. Having understood that, I started adding white chestnut to my remedy. This addition helped me bounce back much faster.

The best thing about this philosophy is a better self-knowledge. Knowing myself is an intrinsic part of my life, and every day that makes me better than what I was yesterday.

INDIAN FLOWER ESSENCES

My faith in Bach flower remedies egged me on to research other flower remedies. From ancient Egypt to modern Australia, flower waters/essences have been used and continue to be made and consumed for their healing properties. In fact, I wouldn't be too wide off the mark if I say that almost every country, culture and tradition, in some form or another, is using the energy and life force of flower-induced waters.

WHAT IS THE INDIAN TRADITION OF FLOWER ESSENCES?

I discussed the subject with Ayurvedic physician Dr Ipsita Chatterjee. It was not much of a surprise to realize that India is a pioneer, of sorts, of healing flower essences. Medicinal waters, traditionally known as '*arkas*' (an ancient Ayurvedic method of making infusions and distillations with flowers, herbs and spices), include a few floral distillations as well. These infusions/concoctions/distillations are perhaps some of the oldest variety of flower essences that are made and consumed to date. In fact, what fascinates me the most about these arkas is the interesting facts and anecdotes associated with them. For instance, do you know who the inventor of arka was? It was none other than Ravana—yes, from Ramayana. In fact, the book *Arka Prakash* is a dialogue between him and his consort Mandodari, wherein he explains the various types of arka, their uses and the process of making them.

Arkas are generally made from spices and herbs, but the book also mentions some floral varieties. In Pushpa Ayurveda, a branch of Ayurveda that focuses on healing with flowers, there's a detailed description of different methods by which flowers could be consumed for medicinal purposes. Among them *pushpa hima* (flower essence made by soaking flowers in water for twelve hours), *pushpa arka* (distilled extract of flowers) and *pushpa sura* (tincture of flowers) are 'floral remedies' that can be considered to be similar to modern-day flower essences.

NEW-AGE INDIAN FLOWER ESSENCES

One of the proponents of contemporary Indian flower essences is Dr Malti Khaitan. Her journey in flower remedies began with her knowledge and practice of Bach flower remedies. In the preface to her book *Flowers That Heal*, Dr Khaitan writes, 'Sharing my knowledge of Bach flower remedies . . . has been my main aim.' This is a sentiment that's very close to Dr Bach's own intent of developing his system of healing with flowers. His desire was to create a simple therapy, which anyone could access to heal themselves. And that's the reason why his system is so focused and compact.

It's true that there is no emotion under the sun that a combination of Dr Bach's repertoire of thirty-eight flower remedies can't address. However, their drawback is that these are essences of European flowers—and, therefore, the need for indigenous flower essences.

Having said that, I feel if the original intent of Dr Bach has to be honoured—that is, a simple system of healing which anyone can benefit from—then based on his methodology, local flowers need to be tapped into for their benefits. Hence, it's important to familiarize ourselves with the existing Indian flower essences and nurture them.

DECODING DR KHAITAN'S LIST OF FLOWERS THAT HEAL

The list below is aimed at providing a brief overview of the remedies. Dr Khaitan's own 'at-a-glance' chart—which is there in her book—was a little confusing for me. So for my better understanding, I have made a few amends and drawn up this list that works as a ready reckoner.

Aloe vera—exhaustion due to work
Amaltas—fear of one's own anger
Ashoka—deep sorrow or grief; female infertility
Ashwagandha—feeling unsettled and unsteady; nervousness leading to insomnia
Asparagus—passivity, despondency and defeatism; female infertility
Balsam—over-concern towards others
Banana—lack of communication skills; fragile bones
Basil—indecision regarding two alternatives; mental exhaustion over decision-making
Bottle brush—extreme anxiety and a deep foreboding about the future
Bougainvillea—low self-esteem; sense of guilt for no reason

Bur—inner disharmony and lack of purpose

Calendula (different from marigold or Indian geinda)—bitterness; ill temper, especially in the manner of speaking

California poppy—attraction towards superficial spirituality, glamour and fame

Canna—unwanted thoughts; constant mental chatter leading to exhaustion and lack of sleep

Celery—nervousness, insomnia and debility

Chamomile—indecisive, irritable, moody, hyperactive and volatile temper

Champa (not frangipani, but the yellow champak or magnolia)—subservience; weakness of will and difficulty of saying no

Coriander—high strung and in pain

Corn—disorientation in an urban setup; preference to be close to nature

Cosmos—lack of focus and clarity; inability to think and communicate clearly

Curry leaf—confusion, nervousness and loneliness

Drumstick—bitterness, resentment

Eucalyptus—claustrophobia and fear of being alone

Feverfew—fretting, touchiness and sudden fits of anger and hysteria

French marigold—slow-learning, repeating mistakes

Geinda—inability to adjust and release emotions

Garlic—fear of something known and specific that drains emotionally

Geranium—unhappiness with life and circumstances

Ginger—shock from traumas like death, accident, divorce, accident or illness

Gooseberry—attention-seeking; craving for love and inability to adjust to others' views and life changes

Grapefruit—stress and taut nerves

Gulmohar—acts of sexual violence

Harshingar—rigidness, perfectionism and unwillingness to change

Hibiscus—deep sense of hopelessness; (in women) a lack of connection with sexuality

Him water (note: This is not a flower water but water from the Ganga)—undue personal meticulousness and unreasonable zeal for 'doing the right thing without harming others'

Hollyhock—lack of trust and difficulty in making commitments

Jasmine—working and functioning better at night, but a drained feeling during the day; connecting better with the Supreme

Kachnaar—feeling insecure and unable to let go of the past

Kadam—emotions clouding reason and logic

Lemon—clouded thoughts and inability to think clearly

Lotus—disharmony, obsessions, misunderstanding, negativity and emotional blocks

Luffa—tendency to break or disregard rules, hyperkinetic children

Mogra; bela—indecision; tonic for feeding mothers

Marjoram—fear of being alone and vulnerable

Morning glory—careless, erratic lifestyle and a susceptibility to addictions

Mulberry—prejudice; feeling of jealousy and hatred

Mustard (similar to the Bach flower remedy of mustard)—
    sudden feeling of gloom for no particular reason
Nasturtium—feeling of being emotionally and intellectually
    drained due to overthinking
Neem—difficulty of focusing in the here and now
Onion—suffering from (the result of) domestic violence
Oregano—inability to understand the body's needs
Ox-eye daisy—lack of clarity and inability to see through
    things
Pansy—deep grief over loss of a loved one; broken heart
Papaya—lack of understanding with partner
Passion flower—lacks tolerance and sensitivity towards
    others' beliefs
Peach—depression and grief; moodiness
Peepal—delusional fears and susceptibility to superstitions
Peppermint—oscillation between two options
Periwinkle—impatience, impulsive behaviour and irritability
Petunia—mischief and hyperactivity
Pine—negative self-image and a consuming sense of guilt
Pomegranate—emotional insecurity and lack of confidence
    (especially in women)
Poppy red—daydreaming, tendency to live in the world of
    imaginations
Portulaca—exhaustion due to stress at work
Radish—feeling of being overwhelmed by life's challenges;
    difficulty in coping with circumstances
Rangoon creeper—vulnerability to others' influence
Red rose—demands love
Salvia—obsession with cleanliness; house pride
Saunf—disharmony in body and mind

Snapdragon—misdirected libido, leading to abusive, aggressive and destructive behaviour

Sunflower—aggressive nature; controlling behaviour

Sweetpea—wandering; inability to form bonds with family, community and society

Tamarind—talkativeness; self-absorbed and over-concerned with one's own problems

Tuberose—exhaustion from being involved in too many things

Walnut (similar to the Bach flower remedy of walnut)—difficulty in adjusting to changes in the environment

Watermelon—lack of physical energy

White poppy—insomnia

White rose—lack of refinement or social grace

Willow (similar to the Bach flower remedy of willow)—self-pity; tendency to think 'why me?'

Yarrow—mind influenced by people, and body affected by climate

Zinnia—lack of joy and laughter in life

Rescue Remedy (much like Rescue Remedy by Dr Bach, this mix by Dr Khaitan is composed of five Indian flower remedies—ashoka, bottle brush, periwinkle, poppy red and peepal—that are very similar to the five Bach flower remedies in terms of their properties)—crisis and emergency situation

Choosing remedies from this list can be a bit of a challenge. However, the only way of learning/mastering that would be by regularly studying the properties and benefits of these remedies and consuming them. Dr Khaitan's daughter,

Shreerupa Khaitan, is in the process of simplifying the remedy repertoire as well as designing courses. Hopefully, once that's accomplished, understanding and accessing Indian flower remedies will become much easier.

CONTEMPORARY FLOWER ESSENCES

Apart from Dr Khaitan there are others like Dr Atul Shah and Dr Rupa Shah, who have done and are continuing to work on creating essences of Indian flowers. Drs Shah's inventory—Aum Himalaya—includes fifty-one flower remedies. Many of these are common and similar in function to Dr Khaitan's remedies. One can get an understanding and purchase Aum Himalaya Flower Essences from www.aumhimalaya.com. The website offers a comprehensive list of the flowers and their use. There are several other practitioners who are working on Indian, specifically Himalayan, flowers to create flower remedies.

One of the most interesting ones is by Tanamaya from Australia. In the 1990s Tanamaya had spent a considerable amount of time in the Himalayas. He explains in his website—www.himalaya.com.au—that while exploring the mountains and the valleys, 'the flowers began speaking to me'. From this life-changing encounter he developed his range of twenty-one 'Himalayan flower enhancers'. He refers to them as 'enhancers' because he believes they are not remedies to correct the 'wrongs' in a person, but their intention is to 'enhance' what is intrinsically 'right' in the individual.

CAN WE MAKE OUR OWN FLOWER ESSENCES?

This is a question that quite naturally arises in our minds. In my home, sourcing flowers, from my garden or local market, can I make my own flower remedies/essences/enhancers? The flowers and my mind seem to say, 'Why not?' Hence, nudged by that thought, I have experimented with some easily accessible flowers like desi gulab, geinda, hibiscus, bela, rajnigandha and *goloncho* (frangipani) to create flower waters. I am not sure whether they really worked or it was a placebo effect, but what I can definitely say is that making these floral waters and consuming them were indeed a happy experience. And why wouldn't they be? Think about it, imagine it . . . You select bright fresh blooms from your little garden, you gently wash them, then immerse the flowers in a jar of water and leave it for a few hours. Then you strain out the flowers and drink that infused water through the day. Isn't that a luxury, an indulgence? Now add some more elements to the process:

1) Look at the flowers and observe your mind. See which flower attracts you.
2) Pick that flower with a heart of gratitude. In fact, say thank you to the flower.
3) Choose your favourite jar or bottle to infuse the flowers in water.
4) Keep it close to the window so that it gets the sunlight or the moonbeams for some hours. You could even play some music or chant to it.

5) Strain out the soaked flowers, make a paste with them and apply on your face as a pack.

6) Finally, take a sip from that flower-infused water and meditate on it. Observe your mind, body and emotions.

If you were to follow this little ritual, I am sure, like me, you too would come out 'enhanced' from the experience.

TIPS ON GETTING STARTED

To begin with, observe flowers either in their natural habitat or your home. It's a good idea to meditate on the blooms that appeal to you. Don't get intimidated at the idea of meditating. Meditation is quite a simple act. It's as simple as just observing your breath or, in the context of this book, just looking at a flower. Draw energy from the flowers and send them your gratitude and love. The intent with which you approach flowers goes a long way in creating their essences.

After you have picked your flowers, the next step is infusing them in mineral water. Dr Bach's remedies employ two methods of infusion. For delicate and fragile blooms, the 'sun' method is practised. This involves floating the flower heads in clean, clear water for three hours in direct sunlight.

Sturdier, woodier plants, and those that bloom when the sun is weak, are prepared by the 'boiling' method, which involves boiling the flowering parts of the plant for half an hour in pure water.

In both cases, once heat has transferred the energy in the flowers to the water, the flowers are strained out and the energized water is mixed with an equal quantity of brandy. This mix is the mother tincture.

One can follow Dr Bach's methodology for creating one's own remedies, but one could also try other methods of energizing the flower waters. For instance, instead of keeping the flowers in the sun, the blooms can be floated in a jar of pure water and left under moonlight. I like to do this with night blooms like bela and *raatkiraani* (queen of the night). The entire process is almost like poetry and I feel it's a method more suited to my temperament. However, I do boil the flowers in water to ensure that the water is suitable for consumption. I don't mix brandy to this, and I just use the water for drinking through the next day. At a time I make only about one litre of flower water.

To prepare remedies, you can subject the infusions to music and/or chants. And you may also add brandy or vodka to preserve them. I did it once and gave it to a few adventurous friends to try.

OBSERVATIONS ON TAKING PERSONAL REMEDIES

Personally, I felt energized and cheerful after taking geinda. Gulab promoted a sense of overall well-being and made me more tolerant. I was able to accept others just as they are. A friend who took bela for ten days felt that she was able to let go of deep-seated hurts and pains; she also felt hibiscus or jaba helped her in feeling grounded. Another friend, who is a yoga practitioner, felt frangipani or goloncho helped her in her meditative practices.

PART 3

SCENTS & SENSUALITY

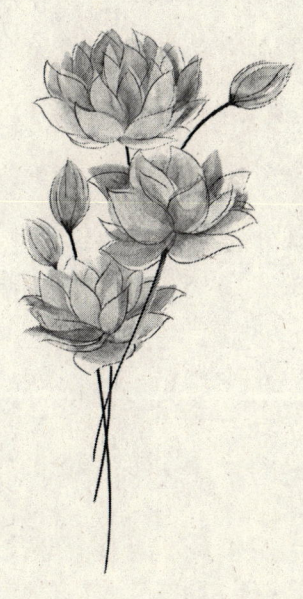

THE FRAGRANT APPEAL OF FLOWERS

What's the first thing that attracts us to a flower? It could be its pretty form, the vibrant colours or the delicateness of its petals. However, even before we see the flower, what may draw us to it is its scent? While almost everything around us—natural or synthetic—has some sort of a smell, it is the smell of flowers that has a more universal appeal. Hence, it is not surprising that most perfumes have a 'floral' note or accord at the heart of its composition.

Indeed, perfumes are like songs. They are compositions like melodies and their 'notes' can be compared to the lyrics of a song. In fact, I feel that while flowers cannot be 'heard' by our physical ears, it is through their fragrances that their enchanting stories are told. To understand more about 'floral' fragrances, let's first take a quick overview of the history of perfumery.

THE FRAGRANT HISTORY

Fragrances and their healing abilities are not a contemporary practice or discovery. It is an ancient art that can be traced back to the annals of most civilizations. In India there's mention of perfumery in texts like *Brihat Samhita*, *Chakra Samhita*, *Gandhayukti* and, of course, *Kama Sutra*. There are relics from the Indus Valley Civilization that include earthen units of perfume distillation. Scents find mention in Egyptian, Persian and Chinese civilizations and, among others, in the Bible. However, the oldest recorded evidence comes from Mesopotamia. What's to be highlighted is that, everywhere, scents were not just adornment. Almost always, they were used for their therapeutic and healing powers.

Another fascinating point about smells is that scents have always been seen as tools of attraction and seduction, and that carries on to date in popular culture. This goes on to corroborate the point that smell is indeed primordial and instinctive. Hence, the hypothesis that kissing is an evolved act of sniffing seems plausible.

THE FIRST PERFUMER

For me the most intriguing aspect of perfume history is what the women contributed to it. The first of that lot, of course being the foremost perfumer of the world, was an alchemist called Tapputi from Mesopotamia. However, there are but just two things we know of her. One, she was the overseer of the royal palace; and, two, she was a perfumer who blended flower oils with calamus (a plant close to lemongrass), myrrh, balsam and cypress, in water or other solvents, and distilled and filtered them to create fragrances.

THE CLEOPATRAS OF THE FRAGRANT WORLD

Cleopatra the Alchemist (not to be confused with Cleopatra the Queen of Egypt), Mary Magdalene, Empress Nur Jahan and Marguerite Maury intrigue me as much as Tapputi does. Cleopatra the Alchemist is said to be one of the four female alchemists—the other three being Mary the Jewess, Madera and Taphnutia—who had discovered the Philosopher's Stone, which is reported to have the ability to create gold out of base metals. Though there is no record of her life and death, it is believed that she was active in Alexandria during the third or fourth century.

Like with her, information, if at all any, regarding the other three women of the quartet is sketchy. In the history of perfumery, Cleopatra the Alchemist is credited for her discovery of the alembic—an apparatus that helps in sublimation and distillation.

A prototype of this alembic is still used in Kannauj, an ancient small town in Uttar Pradesh known for making attars, called the 'Grasse of India'. Tucked in the hills north of Cannes, Grasse has been known as the perfume capital of the world since the sixteenth century.

Incidentally, Cleopatra's contemporary Mary of Jewess is credited for a similar apparatus. In fact, the identities of Cleopatra the Alchemist and Mary of Jewess seem like an amalgamation of several women. For instance, Cleopatra the Alchemist is often referred to as Cleopatra the Physician, but a counter-argument goes that Cleopatra the Physician and Cleopatra the Alchemist were two different individuals and Cleopatra the Alchemist used the name 'Cleopatra' as a pseudonym.

These debates and conjectures make one wonder whether some of the myths and lores surrounding the Egyptian queen Cleopatra could perhaps have been attributed to her equally fascinating namesakes. After all, Cleopatra is legendary for her beauty rituals and especially her fascination with fragrant essential oils of rose and blue lotus. Perhaps her fragrant exploits were actually achievements and discoveries of the other two Cleopatras which were attributed to her, by herself or her entourage, to further her charm and charisma.

Whether or not the queen appropriated the achievements of her contemporaries, it is undeniable that her fragrant stories are stuff that dreams are made of. One of the popular legends claims that Cleopatra had slicked the sails of her ships with neroli essential oil and washed and packed her cedarwood ship with rose water and rose petals respectively. All this was, of course, to seduce Mark Anthony. Hence, it is no wonder that history took the turn that it did. After all, which man could have resisted this glorious indulgence of senses? They say that the way to a man's heart is through his stomach; I say it is through his nose!

Another exotic floral essential that is considered to be Cleopatra's favourite is the blue lotus. The scent of blue lotus is intriguing and intoxicating and is hence referred to as the 'cannabis of ancient Egypt'. It is believed Cleopatra wore the aromatic oil as a fragrance and the Egyptians infused it in their wines.

With these charming weapons, it is no doubt that Cleopatra killed it softly, but have you wondered what effect it could have had on her? A woman who was so skilled in the nuances of sensuality would definitely have to be a woman of strength—a woman who believed in herself. A woman who was well aware of herself—I believe that's what made Cleopatra one of the sexiest women in history.

Inspired by this fascinating woman, on days that I want to assure myself that I deserve only the best in life, I put a drop of desi gulab oil at the centre of my chest, a dab of neroli essential oil on my throat and, finally, I anoint the point between the brows with blue lotus aroma oil.

MARY MARY QUITE CONTRARY

Mary Magdalene is a woman from history who fascinates me with her gentleness and intrigue. Sometimes she is seen as a maudlin disciple of Jesus weeping at his feet. In fact, the word 'maudlin' owes its existence to the sentimentality of Mary Magdalene. She is also seen as repentant sinner, a prostitute who was 'saved' by Jesus and, therefore, eternally devoted to him. Alternative interpretations of the Bible view her as the most trusted disciple of Jesus and his 'closest companion'. Popular culture believes her to be the wife of Jesus. What draws me to her is how her personality is open to such diverse interpretations. And the most fascinating aspect of her life— her association with essential oils.

According to Biblical references, when Jesus was nailed to the cross, Mary anointed his feet with her tears and expensive oil of 'nard' or spikenard—a plant known as *jatamansi* that grows abundantly in the Himalayas and has miraculous healing properties. It is believed that after Jesus's crucifixion, Mary travelled to France and lived there for another thirty years where she worked as a healer using essential oils and poultices. Theologians like Holger Kersten and Nicolas Notovich, and groups like Ahmadiyya founded by Mirza Ghulam Ahmad, believe that Jesus did not die on the cross; rather he and a certain 'Mary' escaped and travelled to India, where they lived in Kashmir for many years. The controversial Rozabal shrine in Srinagar is believed to be the tomb of Jesus. My imaginative mind and romantic soul are inclined to believe this fascinating story of Jesus and Mary Magdalene. I feel this supposition also in some way could explain how Mary came to possess the jatamansi oil from India . . . perhaps she did have a connection with India.

Apart from the jatamansi, Mary is often associated with other essential oils of rose, jasmine, frankincense and myrrh. In fact, there are some perfumes and oil blends named 'Mary Magdalene', which contain these essential oils or extracts and are composed following Ayurvedic tradition. Some of them are specifically used for Indian meditation practices like kundalini awakening.

To strengthen my root chakra, let go of hurts and open my heart and mind to universal love and wisdom, I often use a blend of desi gulab, mogra, Kashmiri lavender and jatamansi. In a 10 ml roll-on bottle, I put two drops of each of these essential oils and fill the rest of the bottle with sweet almond oil. I apply this oil on my pulse points before meditating.

Before moving ahead to the next woman of the fragrance world, let's just reflect a while on the popular nursery rhyme:

Mary, Mary, quite contrary,
how does your garden grow?
With silver bells, and cockle shells,
and pretty maids all in a row.

Like other nursery rhymes, this one too has religious and historical allegory. Interpreters of the rhyme have seen the 'Mary' of the poem as Mother Mary; Mary, Queen of Scots; and Mary I of England. However, I feel this poem could also allude to Mary Magdalene. Controversial Mary, her garden of flowers and herbs . . . all this could very well be references to Mary Magdalene, no?

ANOTHER MAURY OF AROMATHERAPY

Rene Gattefosse, a French chemist, who accidentally burnt his hand while working in the laboratory, is said to be the pioneer of modern aromatherapy. When he scalded his hand he plunged it into a jar containing lavender oil. This not only healed his wounds but spurred him on to experiment more with essential oils and their therapeutic values. In 1928 he coined the word 'aromatherapie' and this marked the arrival of what we know today as aromatherapy. This is what I call turning poison into medicine, where an accident led to the discovery of the finest healing anointment.

Dr Jean Valet took this therapy ahead and used it for healing burns and wounds of soldiers injured during the First World War. He also successfully treated psychological ailments with essential oils, thereby establishing aroma oils' power of healing physically, physiologically and psychologically. However, the person credited to have pioneered the use of essential oils in beauty therapy was an Austrian-born biochemist, Madam Marguerite Maury. While she was working with a surgeon in Alsace, she read a book called *Les Grandes Possibilités par les Matières Odoriferantes*

(The Great Possibilities of Aromatic Substances) by Dr Chabenes, written in 1838. Incidentally, he was also the teacher of Gattefosse. The book became Maury's guide and set her on her journey with aromatherapy. In 1961 she wrote a book *Le Capital Jeunesse*; however, the book did not receive the attention it deserved. In 1964 it was released in Britain under the title *The Secret of Life and Youth* and it remains a sort of bible for contemporary aromatherapy.

Through her years of research and practical application, Maury developed a unique form of massage using blends of essential oils. Her entire work—choice and use of essential oils and massage—was based solely on the principles that we can remain youthful in our attitude, energies and beliefs if we keep our systems clear and functioning effectively. This, she believed, could be achieved by practising aromatherapy. Maury lectured and gave seminars on the subject throughout Europe and opened aromatherapy clinics in Paris, Switzerland and England.

She possessed some of the eccentricities of a genius, but she was also a generous and loveable woman, and a magnetic and charismatic person. She was a whirlwind of energy and enthusiasm, working ceaselessly till the day she breathed her last. Her last manuscript, found at her bedside, began with the words, 'The aromatherapy involved in cosmetology can lead to the most extraordinary of results.'

FEAST OF FRESH FLOWERS

I believe fragrances from flowers and their benefits in our lives can be categorized into three groups—scent of fresh flowers, aromas of floral essential oils and floral perfumes. While fresh flowers are primarily worn for their visual beauty, as hair adornments or accessories, some flowers are specifically worn for their fragrance. For instance, jasmine or mogra or jui is mostly worn for their heady notes. Some fragrant flowers are grown in homes or kept in living spaces in order to fragrance the area. Raatkiraani, *hasnuhana*, parijaat, kadam, keya, bela, mogra, gulab, golden champak and rajnigandha are planted around homes and in house gardens for their beautiful aromas.

My maternal grandmother would place little bowls of water with fresh bela or golden champak flowers in different rooms of the house. Inspired by her, I continue this practice of placing bowls with flowers around my home and workplace. The gentle aromas fill the spaces and soothe the mind and soul. While I extensively use fresh seasonal flowers, like geinda, bela, champak, shiuli, rajnigandha and nargis, my heart skips a beat when it comes to the petals of the desi gulab.

LEGEND OF THE ROSE

Once, for a dinner I hosted in my home, I created a small bed of gulab petals at the centre of the table and placed a few candles on it. As the evening grew, the aroma of the gulab opened up and hung around the rooms like a fragrant, invisible cloud.

My favourite way of using gulab as a fragrance is by using it as a mouth freshener. In a petal I place an elaichi and a *laung* (interestingly, this spice is a flower) along with a few grains of saunf. This combination creates an explosion of flavours and fragrances in the mouth.

Here, I must say my love for the gulab is inspired by the Mughal queen Mehrunisa (known popularly as Nur Jahan).

As the story goes, Mehrunisa's fiery temper was as legendary as her passionate love for Jehangir. Once the royal couple had a public altercation, where Mehrunisa flew into a rage and slapped the emperor. This, everyone thought, was the end of Mehrunisa. However, soon Jehangir announced a ceremony for which the pathway of the palace garden was strewn with rose petals. At a particular time when the sunrays fell on the petals and they let out their robust smell, Mehrunisa walked from one end of the pathway, Jehangir from the other end, and they met midway, in that haze of red and intoxicating fragrance. I read about this for the first time in the historical novel *A Feast of Roses* by Indu Sunderesan, which is based on the life and love of Jehangir and Mehrunisa. There are several versions and interpretations of this story I have come across in this book.

Incidentally, stories and tales also indicate that the rose essential oil was accidentally discovered in India by Mehrunisa. According to the records of Italian traveller Niccolao Manucci, who lived in the Mughal palace during Jehangir's reign, the rose essential oil was discovered by Mehrunisa. The empress discovered it while bathing in the Shahi Hamam (royal baths), when she noticed an oily film in the water from rose petals left overnight.

However, according to Jehangir himself, in his autobiographical work, *Tuzuki Jehangiri* (Memories of Jehangir), once Asmat Begam (Mehrunisa's mother, who was known for her skill of making fragrant water) was making rose water when she noticed a thick mass on the surface of pots where hot rose water had been poured from jugs. She collected this 'oily' layer and realized that it was so fragrant that a single drop of it rubbed on to the palm filled the air with an enchanting scent of tonnes of red roses blooming simultaneously. Jehangir was so charmed by this delightful fragrance that he presented Asmat with a pearl necklace. It is believed that Emperor Akbar's wife Salima Begam named this essential oil 'Jehangiri attar'— 'Jehangir's perfume'.

HEALING AROMATIC OILS

What shall I say of essential oils? Well, let me put it this way—if you haven't experienced them, you have not truly lived your life, as yet. No, I am not being dramatic. I honestly believe that using aromatic oils transforms your life physically, psychologically and spiritually. My encounter with essential oils happened quite early (when I was about ten to twelve years old), courtesy of my mother, who is an aesthetician and a make-up artist. After doing a course in aromatherapy, she introduced in our home small, fragrant bottles of oils. I took to these like fish to water. I discarded my 'deos' and started putting in drops of lavender, rose, orange and lemon essential oils in my bath water. I loved the subtle aroma they would leave on my skin and how they made me feel no less than Cleopatra. For a shy girl, this indulgent experience was not just a 'feel-good' practice, it was an empowering ritual.

WHAT ARE ESSENTIAL OILS?

Essential oils are aromatic, concentrated, hydrophobic liquids that are extracted from plants. They contain numerous, complex compounds like terpenes, esters, aldehydes, ketones, alcohols, phenols and oxides, which make them highly therapeutic. Unlike fixed or fatty oils, essential oils are extremely *volatile* and, therefore, quickly evaporate when exposed to air. Some of these oils like lavender, rosemary, pine, lemon and basil are watery or alcohol-like in texture, while oils of myrrh, benzoin and vetiver can be viscous and sticky.

HOW ESSENTIAL ARE ESSENTIAL OILS?

The reason these aromatic oils are called 'essential' is because they contain the 'essence' of the plant's fragrance and its therapeutic property. 'Essential' in case of these oils does not necessarily mean 'indispensable' as with the terms 'essential amino acid' or 'essential fatty acid', which are so called because they are nutritionally required by a living organism. However, I feel the benefits of these compounds will not be duly respected or, for that matter, properly tapped if we don't start giving them the status of being 'indispensable' in our daily lives.

I can only speak for myself, and I feel that my life has completely transformed—making me stronger and younger in mind and body—with essential oils. I experienced their immense healing potential and beauty while doing my course in aromatherapy from Dr Ravi Ratan. During a class, I had developed severe stomach ache. It was an excruciating pain in my lower abdomen, which I had been experiencing for a few months but had not really been able to understand what was causing it. Dr Ratan asked me to immediately apply lavender oil on my stomach and smell it. Miraculously, the pain disappeared within a few minutes and I was also feeling a lot more relaxed.

Later during the same course, I had a sudden bout of coughing. Again Dr Ratan handed me a little bottle of oil and asked me to have a drop of it. It was a pungent, sharp blend and, yet again, almost instantly it stopped my coughing. Through the course, several health and emotional issues kept surfacing. With different aroma oils, via inhalation, topical application and internal consumption, I started understanding my body, mind and soul. This had been a rather challenging but fulfilling experience. The sudden overflow of suppressed emotions were overwhelming, but it also helped me accept myself as I am and then gently improve myself little by little each day.

HEALING ME SOFTLY

While I work with all types of essential oils, like oils from roots, stems, spices, leaves, fruits and flowers, I am more inclined towards floral essential oils as they appeal to my soul. Dr Ratan believes that different categories of essential oils address different groups of issues. For instance, root oils like vetiver, *patchouli* and jatamansi help in grounding and physically improving bone health and strengthening connective tissue. Similarly, he explains that citrus oils like orange, lemon, bergamot and tangerine help clear throat ailments as well as promote better expression and communication. I agree with this view and I make different blends with all categories of essential oils; however, I feel essential oils of flowers can address all emotional issues. And that's why all my blends of Jhelum Loves Bach & Aroma remedies have at least one or two floral essential oils.

AROMA MANTRA

There are numerous aromatic oils from flowers; however, the ones I use frequently and extensively are lavender, gulab, geranium, mogra, neroli and blue lotus.

'Lavender Dreams'

The hills come alive
with the purple haze.
The scented breeze
sings a soulful song
that soothes the bruised heart.
At sundown
a flower witch sits by her window
with a glass of pearly wine.
In it she has added
two drops of lavender,
a sprig of rosemary,
a drop of lime.
She sips her potent drink,
remembers the little girl,
who no longer returns with the horses
from the lavender fields.

She lights a candle
made of frankincense and myrrh,
floats four strands of saffron
in a silver bowl of warm milk.
Next to it, she places an amethyst
washed in the flowing waters of the Jhelum.
Energized thereafter,
with four drops of Kashmiri lavender,
and with hope in her eyes,
she whispers a spell:

O moonbeams peeking through the clouds,
bathe these pine forests and lavender fields
with your gentle shower of love.
Take my prayer to every corner of this universe;
bring heaven back to where it belongs.

Lavender is a saviour of sorts and is one of the few essential oils that can be applied directly on the skin without diluting it in a carrier oil (like olive, jojoba or coconut oils) or water. If you had to pick just one essential oil for your life, then lavender would surely qualify for the spot. The most versatile of all essential oils, lavender has clean, fresh, floral top notes and subtle, herbaceous undertones. It is antiseptic, analgesic, anti-allergic and an excellent healer. Plus, it has a warm soothing aroma that makes it an ideal single-note perfume for daily wear. I keep a bottle of lavender in my room, in my bag and also in office for emergency and first aid. Massage a few drops of lavender and white chestnut Bach flower remedy for good, revitalizing sleep.

The purple bloom thrives at 3000 feet above sea level and one of the finest qualities used to be produced in France. However, in recent years, Kashmiri lavender has amassed huge popularity and is now sought after internationally. This Indian variety is slightly more bitter and astringent than its European counterparts. You can even try growing it in your kitchen garden. Just ensure that it gets good sunlight and water doesn't stagnate around it. Ideally, you should just sprinkle water on it.

MYTH AND MAGIC

There are several legends and ancient practices that link lavender to peace, healing and well-being. When Adam and Eve were ordered out of Eden, they apparently carried only a lavender plant with them. Another biblical story reveals that the lavender got its lovely fragrance only after Mother Mary set out Baby Jesus's clothes to dry on a lavender plant. And among other floral essential oils, Cleopatra also used lavender to seduce Julius Caesar and Mark Anthony. However, what fascinates me most about lavender is the dream interpretations of the flower and magic that has got associated with it. It is believed that dreaming of lavender is an indication of good luck and prosperity. The essential oil is also supposed to increase clairvoyance and, therefore, has often been used for meditation and dreamwork.

MOOD LIFTER

The plant has such a powerful impact that when you are depressed, if you just gaze at the lavender fields, your mood will be lifted. If you cannot take yourself to a lavender field, follow this simple visualization. At a quiet place, sit and look at a picture of lavender fields. You can also play a santoor track while you practise this. Choose a five- to ten-minute piece as that's all that you need for this meditation. Take a drop of the essential oil in your palms and inhale. Take a couple of deep breaths and then focus on your breathing. Think of the beautiful valleys of Kashmir and imagine them enveloped in a purple haze. This little exercise will uplift your emotions, help control mood swings and balance the chakras.

SKIN SALVE

The antiseptic, anti-inflammatory and anti-fungal properties of this wonder oil make it my first choice for beauty blends. It fights acne, inhibits bacteria that can lead to infection-causing breakouts, heals skin and helps in treating scars.

Just a couple of days before my engagement, I had gone to a salon for a face clean-up and some peel that they used had burnt my skin. I rushed home and immediately applied aloe vera gel and lavender oil on the affected area. Every two hours I kept applying this mix and by next morning the redness had gone, but the skin was starting to peel. Then I switched to applying pure coconut oil with a few drops of lavender. By next evening my skin had healed completely and there was no scar mark!

STRESS BUSTER

Stress and tension are major problems in today's world and using lavender oil to relieve these symptoms can help. Sniffing the essential oil frequently or adding a few drops in your bathing water alleviates stress, anxiety and depression. A drop or two of lavender and clary sage oils on your pillow are an effective remedy for insomnia.

PAIN SLAYER

Lavender has the ability to relax tensed nerves and that is the reason why it can reduce headaches and migraines. Take a few drops of lavender oil and massage it on your lower abdomen for 5–10 minutes to tackle menstrual cramps. Other than relieving pain, the oil has a psychological effect on the mood swings that you experience during periods.

'Romancing the Rose'

After her evening bath
with the oil of rose,
she anoints her brow and heart.
On the floor she draws a circle
with petals of nine desi gulabs
and then steps into the ring,
armed with a photograph
and a flaming rose in hand.

As the sun mellows,
and moon swells,
Spirit of Love,
protect and keep together,
me and my soulmate.

Illuminate our home
with a rosy glow;
may joy, peace and hope overflow.

On Friday nights,
when the stars shine bright,
the flower witch
casts her spell thrice.

Rose otto is one of the most exquisite-smelling oils and is almost always seen as a symbol of love and passion. Perhaps because it addresses the sweetest human emotion, this coveted oil also has numerous physical and psychological benefits.

Relaxing, uplifting, aphrodisiacal and healing, rose essential oil is one of my favourite natural ingredients. The essential oil of rose has a frequency of 350 MHz and, therefore when we apply it, it also raises our frequency. As a part of skincare, it heals, rejuvenates and nourishes skin. It is especially good for matured skin and can also be used as an eye wash. And when applied at the centre of the chest, it opens and balances the heart chakra and thereby inspires courage and compassion.

TYPES OF ROSE OILS

Rose oil is the essential oil extracted from the petals of different types of rose. There are two varieties of rose oils based on their method of extraction—rose otto, which is extracted by steam distillation, and rose absolute, which is obtained through solvent extraction, the absolute being used more commonly in perfumery. While the benefits of the two oils are almost similar, rose otto is more expensive than rose absolute because a larger quantity of rose petals is required to extract the oil by this method. Rose absolute is more viscous and darker than rose otto, and most perfumers prefer it because rose absolute's smell is closer to the smell of the actual flower.

SPICY ROSE

The Indian rose oil or the rooh gulab (means the soul of rose) is traditionally extracted by the steam distillation method. I use this oil extensively in making my skincare and fragrance blends. It is indeed the fragrance of the soul. There is something magical about the robust peppery note of the desi gulab. This spark comes from eugenol, a naturally occurring ingredient in certain essential oils. It is present in high quantities in black pepper essential oil. So if you smell a blend of black pepper in geranium oil (which shares with rose oil a common ingredient, geranium), it will seem a lot like rose. Rooh gulab can be worn as single-note perfume. I also like wearing it in combination with vetiver or khus. My favourite mix is two drops of oud with a drop of desi gulab oil.

GULAB JAL (ROSE WATER)

The petals of gulab are steam-distilled to extract the healing and nourishing rose essential oil. During distillation a by-product is made, which is our all-time favourite beauty staple—gulab jal or rose water, which can be easily made at home by boiling rose petals in water and straining the petals out. The use of rose water goes back centuries, to when Romans used to add petals to their water and wines to connect to the goddess of love, Venus, and when Egyptian queen Cleopatra used it to maintain her beauty. In India, gulab jal is sprinkled to welcome guests during celebrations and when entering shrines.

THE LEGEND

Earlier in this chapter I have shared a couple of myths and legends associated with rose. And these are but just a small sample of the legends of the rose that abound in history. In fact, in whichever land the rose grows, there is sure to be a legend or myth around it. In India, stories and lores of desi gulab abound. My favourite, of course, is the legend of Mehrunisa and Jehangir. But there are a couple of other interesting ones as well. Goddess Lakshmi is always associated with the pink lotus or the *padma*. In fact, Lakshmi's other names like Padma, Padmaja, Kamala and Padmini mean lotus. However, according to legend, Lakshmi was created by Lord Brahma using 108 big roses and 1008 small roses. How beautiful is that?

EMOTIONAL HEALING

The oil is popularly known for its antidepressant qualities, which help in keeping a person mentally strong and confident. When used in aromatherapy, it brings in feelings of glee and promise, and helps in uplifting those with a nervous disposition through its serene bouquet effect.

A gentle massage of rose oil works wonders to reduce menopausal symptoms. Very effective for the immune system, the oil protects our body from various viruses and reduces chances of catching viral infections. Try a blend of 30 ml olive oil with two drops of desi gulab oil and four drops of khus oil.

GLOWING SKIN

Rose essential oil has also been used widely in skin and beauty care. The best way to reap its antiseptic benefits is to add a few drops of the oil into any DIY creams or oil blend. Here's a simple recipe: 30 ml of rosehip oil, 2 drops of rose oil and 4 drops of sandalwood oil.

'Humble Geranium'

Though this ubiquitous, non-demanding bloom
is popularly known as the poor man's rose,
for me, it is not 'poor' at all.
Its rich, complex fragrance
makes it one of my favourite single-note scents.
As a daily wear,
I love rubbing it on my hair,
behind my knees and ears.
If you wish to compose a scent,
here's a recipe to try.
In a large peg of dark rum,
add a drop each of neroli, vanilla, cinnamon.
Throw in four drops of cedarwood oil
and top it up with six drops of geranium.
Pour this scented mix in a glass bottle
and let it rest for two weeks.
Use it then, liberally, as a body mist.

Geranium, like lavender, is an all-rounder. In skincare it is preferred for its cleansing, astringent and balancing properties. Geranium helps balance hormones and, therefore, I like wearing it as perfume to alleviate PMS (premenstrual syndrome). I often use geranium mixed with crab apple and scleranthus Bach flower remedies to create a cleansing and calming face mist.

THE LEGEND

It is believed that once Prophet Mohammed went to the mountain to pray and hung his sweaty shirt on a shrub to dry. When he came back to pick it up, he found it covered with fragrant flowers. That was the birth of geranium. There are several other myths and beliefs surrounding these flowers. One of my favourite stories is that pink geranium was often used for love spells. I am not surprised; its sensuous fragrance can easily create an aura of romance.

ALL THAT IT NEEDS

As I said, geranium is one of the least demanding flowers. In fact, it is hard not to grow it right. The flowers bloom in any soil, love sunshine and need very little water. While geranium grows in many countries, like France, Spain, Italy, Morocco, Egypt and China, one of the best varieties grows in Ooty in south India. In the last couple of years it is being grown in abundance and as a successful commercial crop in Kashmir. Very little is needed to grow these flowers in your balcony, terrace and patio, to add fragrance and colour to your home environment.

ROSE-LIKE

Geranium essential oil contains an ingredient called geraniol that is also present in rose oil. Since some varieties of geranium smell a lot like rose, the essential oil of the plant is often used in formulations to either replace or complement the scent of rose. Geranium is also a great healer for skin and hence it is often used in skincare formulations to get the benefits of rose and to have a 'rose-like' smell.

THE ALL-ROUNDER

Geranium essential oil is antibacterial, antifungal, antispasmodic and a great cleanser. Its fresh, floral, spicy smell, with overtones of citrus makes it a wonderful uplifting scent. Due to these qualities it is extensively used in aromatherapy formulations for skincare, haircare and emotional healing. I use geranium essential oil in most of my Jhelum Loves Bach & Aroma Remedies formulations like Honeytrap face wash, Soothsayer face mist, Divinity face cream, Elixir face oil and Energizer shampoo.

'Mogra Magic'

This balmy summer evening,
I close my eyes
and walk down the lane
of the familiar and fond.
On the way I pick up
the delicate white garland
that I often wear
on my hair.

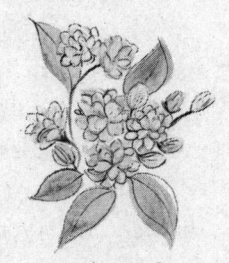

O Sweet Jasmine,
your fragrant nostalgia
pulls at my heartstrings.
It releases hurts of yore
and mends bonds that had torn.

Uplifting, an antidepressant and an aphrodisiac, the scent of mogra or jasmine essential oil evokes nostalgia in me. While, of course, jasmine oil is great for skin and hair rejuvenation, I prefer it more for its aromatic beauty and emotional effect. Born and brought up in north Kolkata—the older part of the city—mogra and its other varieties like bela and jui have been an intrinsic part of my childhood. Bengali New Year, which falls on either 14 or 15 April, marks the entry of these fragrant white blooms in our lives, with women decking their buns, knots and rolls with thick garlands of bela. Through the summer and monsoon these delicate flowers would fill the warm, damp air with their breezy, heady aroma. If you happen to be in Kolkata during monsoons, and if your car stops at a traffic light, do remember to buy a few garlands of jasmine from the flower sellers. It will make your evening fragrant and memorable.

FLORAL ANECDOTES

While jasmine and its brethren are popular all across India, the variety that has created a niche internationally is the Madurai *malligai* (jasmine). In fact, this variety has now been given the GI (geographical indication) tag in 2013.

The Madurai jasmine has several stories and legends associated with it. Among them—the one I find the most fascinating—is the story that Dr Ipsita Chatterjee shared with me about Goddess Meenakshi adorning and anointing herself with these flowers for her union with Lord Sundareswarar. Incidentally, Goddess Meenakshi and Lord Sundareswarar are reincarnations of Shiva and Parvati and the spring festival

Chitirai celebrates their marriage. According to the traditions of this unique nuptial, it is Goddess Meenakshi who receives the hand of Lord Sundareswarar, unlike other customs where the groom receives the hand of the bride.

HEALING EMOTIONS

While jasmine essential oil is excellent for hair and skin care, I am particularly impressed by its effect on the sacral chakra. The sacral or the *swadishthan* chakra is located below the navel and is supposed to be the seat of emotions and sexuality. Hurt, pain, anger, jealousy, lust, sadness and other negative emotions arise when this chakra is blocked. Application of jasmine essential oil at the chakra point helps transform these emotions and can simultaneously help address ailments like uterine fibroids, polycystic ovaries and endometriosis. When used in combination with sandalwood or tea tree oil for sitz baths, it can cure urinary tract infections. The essential oil when smelt or applied behind ears has an instant relaxing effect, which helps relieve stress.

Plus, it has aphrodisiac properties. So if you wish to create your own romantic scent, mix 4 drops of sandalwood essential oil with 2 drops of jasmine oil in 10 ml of jojoba oil, or distilled water or vodka—whichever base you choose. A drop of the essential oil can also be worn as a single-note perfume. My favourite and most indulgent combination is a mix of three exotic flower oils—desi gulab, jasmine and blue lotus. It is a stunning combination. Just a word of caution: Use these precious oils sparingly as the mix can have a slight intoxicating effect.

'Lure of the Lotus'

The *neel kamal* was her favourite flower;
and so on moonless nights she bathed
with the oil of this fragrant bloom.
Then gazing at a lapis lazuli rock,
she writes this spell
with a peacock plume:

Hark, thy indigo night!
Let this intoxicating scent
of the rare neel kamal
bind you tight.
May those who smell it
always remember:
that the darkest hour
gives birth to this wonder.

The lotus flower or the kamal has always fascinated me—a beautiful bloom that blossoms in the murkiest of waters. Its symbolism is profound, and the deeper I delve into Buddhism and chakra therapy to understand it, the more I am intrigued by it. Ancient Hindu and Buddhist writings link the lotus flower to serenity and purity. It is also said to have soothing and calming effects that make it a perfect choice for meditation. Lotus oil is generally viscous and has an intense floral scent with accents of green notes. Lotus oil has now become one of the essential ingredients for manufacturing skin and personal care products like massage oils, bath soaps and body lotions. This exquisite oil is also

used in aromatherapy as its rich fragrance provides a feeling
of peace.

SPIRITUAL SIGNIFICANCE

While the spiritual nuances of lotus may differ from one
religion to another, one belief that is shared by all is that
the lotus symbolizes, even in the murkiest of circumstances,
our ability to remain unstained. It also shows that out of the
worst the best can emerge. Nichiren Daishonin's Buddhism,
which is based on the Lotus Sutra, believes that the lotus
signifies the law of cause and effect because it is the only
flower that blooms and seeds simultaneously. This means
that the moment we create a cause, its effect is simultaneously
initiated. It symbolizes hope, purity and spiritual awakening,
and it is believed that those who practise the Lotus Sutra are
able to muster hope, courage and compassion. According to
one folklore, wherever the Buddha went he left a trail of lotus
flowers, with every step that he took. An interpretation of this
myth might be that the practitioners of the lotus sutra bring
hope and happiness wherever they go.

In Hinduism, the flower is associated with several gods
and goddesses. Most deities are seen holding the flower or
seated on the lotus. In fact, it is believed that Durga Puja is
incomplete without an offering of 108 pink lotuses. Legend
has it that before going to war with Ravan, Ram had wanted
to worship Devi Durga. Since the goddess could be pleased
with an offering of 108 lotus flowers, Ram did his best to
gather these blooms. However, he fell short of one. That's
when Ram prepared to offer his one eye that resembled a blue

lotus to Devi Durga. Impressed by his devotion, the goddess appeared before him and blessed him.

NEEL KAMAL

The kamal essential oil has three variants—blue, pink and white lotus. Of the three, blue lotus is my favourite. It has the most gorgeous fragrance and acts as an antidepressant, thus helping in relieving stress. It also helps improve skin and hair. I use this oil in some of my products like Dreamcatcher Under-eye Oil, Fanaa (Fragrance of Love—a perfume) and Intuition (the oil blend for the third chakra). I have added it to the under-eye oil because it is an excellent antioxidant; it soothes the skin and makes it look fresher and younger. It is an antidepressant and relieves anxiety and stress and therefore it is in the chakra oil.

BEAUTY BENEFITS

Rich in vitamins B and C, iron and protein, this essential oil helps condition hair, and moisturize and improve the texture of the skin. Add a few drops of lotus oil diluted in carrier oils like jojoba, apricot or almond and use it to massage skin or hair.

AROMA OF ENCHANTMENT

Apart from its cosmetic benefits and spiritual significance, what captivates me most is the smell of blue lotus essential oil. I first caught the whiff of it in an aromatherapy and perfumery class. I had never smelt anything like that before. It was sweet, heady and velvety. It was the first time I experienced a scent that can have a tactile effect. It was like a caress—soft yet crackling with a silent intensity. Since that first encounter I have used this essential oil in many ways: primarily as a single-note perfume—just two drops, that's all you need. Anything more can give you a headache.

There's an art to wearing it. First take a drop of the oil on the palm and then, with the ring finger, dab on the brow centre, base of the throat and behind the ears. Then rub the remaining traces on the wrists and run them over the head to gently perfume the tresses.

The blue lotus oil is certainly not an everyday scent. It is best worn in the evening with something classic and empowering. I love pairing it with sarees. And whenever I have worn this perfume I have had people ask—what are you wearing? Now, after an enquiry like that, would you wear anything else but that? And if that's not enough for you, on special evenings, you can make it headier by combining it with a drop of oud or agarwood oil. The two make a deadly, heady combination.

'Neroli Sunshine'

The evergreen tree
bears a bitter fruit,
but it has a sweet-scented bloom—
a delicate flower called neroli.

Honeybees are drawn to its joyous smell,
sad souls seek its nectar.

Bathed in milk and rose,
the flower witch slicks her hair
with the sunny oil of neroli.
She decks her altar
with these white flowers
that illuminate the darkness
of the mind and heart.

Holding a ball of citrine,
she chants this rhyme
before her floral shrine:

Oh winter, as you melt into spring,
let joy and laughter through my home ring.
And may love and hope sing,
always at my door and windowsill.

Neroli essential oil is made by steam-distilling the fragrant white flowers of the bitter orange. The aroma of these delicate blossoms is an enchanting floral and citrusy mix that immediately makes its way to your head and uplifts the mood. It can be a little heady and intoxicating. No wonder the bees encircling these flowers look like they are 'buzzed'.

GOOD TO KNOW

The bitter orange tree produces three distinctly different essential oils. The peel of the fruit yields bitter orange oil; the leaves are the source of petitgrain essential oil, and the waxy flowers of the tree are steam-distilled to obtain neroli essential oil.

Timing is crucial when it comes to creating neroli essential oil since the flowers quickly lose their oil after they are plucked from the tree. To keep the quality and quantity of neroli essential oil at their highest, the orange blossom should be handpicked without bruising the delicate blooms.

WHAT'S IN A NAME?

Neroli oil's aroma has also been associated with royalty and beauty for centuries. Legend has it that the word 'neroli' is derived from the name of the Italian princess of Nerole, Marie Anne de La Trémoille. Neroli was her favourite oil and 'signature' scent. Some myths say that the oil could have got its name after the Roman emperor Nero. Some say that neroli has got its name from the Sanskrit word 'nagarana'.

THE HAPPY OIL

The smell of neroli makes me smile. It's like a breath of sunshine in a dark wintry day. There have been times when I have been feeling low and just a sniff of this oil has refreshed my mind and heart. I believe neroli also helps one express oneself in the right way, the reason why I use it in my blend of throat chakra oil called Express. I often use this blend on my throat when I have a cold or cough, and it has always soothed me.

Neroli is rich in antioxidants and, therefore, it is a great oil to use in skincare products. It kills free radicals, repairs and nourishes skin and reduces pigmentation. It also helps maintain the right oil balance in the skin, making it an excellent choice for all skin types.

However, personally, I love using neroli for its fragrance and the effect it has on other essential oils. Wearing neroli oil can be a bit tricky as just a little extra can make the blend too heady. Many like using neroli as a single-note perfume and to use the essential oil directly on the skin; however, I like to use it in combination with other essential oils or in a carrier oil.

BLENDING AND MIXING

Neroli is quite versatile and mixes well with most essential oils. Its uniqueness is that just a drop of it can transform a blend without really leaving a pronounced trace of itself. Here are a few ways in which I use it:

1) as a scented body oil: neroli oil (1 drop) in jojoba or olive oil (1 tbsp);
2) as a perfume concentrate: sandalwood oil (2 ml) with neroli oil (2 drops);
3) as a body mist: neroli oil (a touch in 60 ml water) in combination with any one (3–4 drops) of geranium, tuberose, jasmine, cedarwood, lavender or blue lotus essential oil;
4) as a perfume: in a 10–15 ml spray bottle, topped up with water or vodka, neroli oil (2 drops) mixed with cedarwood oil (5 ml), vetiver oil (3 ml), lavender (1 ml) and black pepper (2 drops);
5) as a room freshener: vanilla (6 drops) and neroli essential oils (4 drops) in 60 ml of mineral water. Put it in a spray

bottle and shake it to mix it well. Spritz it on yourself, your room and your bed linen.

HOW FRAGRANT IS MY KITTY

Mademoiselle Coco Chanel's statement 'A woman who doesn't wear perfume has no future' may appear a little harsh, but, in being dramatic, it does underscore the importance of fragrances in our lives.

Since my teens I have had an array of scents—essential oils, quaint perfumes, attars as well as regular body mists—to go with different moods, occasions and seasons. I used aromatic oils of orange, rose and lavender in my bathwater; and wore notes from my treasured bottle of Cacharel's Anais Anais for special summer evenings, Davidoff's Cool Water on regular college days and warm accords of Dior's Poison for winter parties. Options were limited then, which is why making a style statement with signature scents was pretty easy.

However, the world of perfumes changed dramatically in the last decade and a half. There has literally been an explosion of sorts. The sheer variety of scents that are now available on the shelf can be intimidating.

Walk into a departmental store and, from the very door, a perfume strip is poked into your nose. Enter an elevator, you may be assailed or welcomed with a sweet or syrupy smell of the previous occupant hanging in the air like a thick, invisible fog. Step into a spa and the strong whiff of lemongrass will invariably be there to knock you out. In this super-scented environment, choosing perfumes and wearing them with a touch of your personal style has become a difficult task indeed.

A FEW OF MY FAVOURITE FUMES

Despite this avalanche, there are some scents—incidentally, they are all floral fragrances—that have stood out for me and grown on me. These, I can say, are my signature scents, perfumes that reflect my personality.

FINDING MY POISON

Dior's Poison was my first encounter with the world of luxury. In 1986 my parents went for a Europe tour, and in those days when you travelled abroad, you got back exquisite bottles of fine fragrances. Ma had come back with a bottle of Poison, and from then on, it became a fragrance that just remained with her. And she continues to be loyal to it to this day.

I grew up seeing my mother wear it on special evenings. Cautiously, she would open the apple-shaped falcon and, with its crystal glass stopper, dab the perfume behind her ears and on her wrists. The heady notes of tuberose, rose, coriander and vanilla would fill the room and trailed her wherever she went. The image of my mother wearing this gorgeous fragrance became a defining moment of beauty for me. Over the years, several variants of Poison have been released, but for my mother, sister and me the 'original' Poison remains a constant in our wardrobe. It is like a legacy—an inheritance of sorts.

Several years later, in 2009, I encountered another creation of Dior that blew me away. It was their India-inspired fragrance, Escale a Pondichéry. The first whiff of the black tea accord, followed by notes of jasmine and cardamom that left a gentle trail of sandalwood, impressed me to the core. It felt as if Poison is night and Pondichéry is day.

It was launched in Pondicherry and journalists across the globe were flown down to India to attend its launch. And in an unforgettable walk through a local flower market, Francoise Demachy, creator of Pondichéry, quipped that this perfume was a 'foreigner's first impression of India'. However, he said Pondichéry was not the brand's first ode to India. Much before, in 1985, Poison used the Indian tuberose as one of its key ingredients. However, sadly, Pondichéry has been discontinued. But to date, on rainy, summer afternoons when I have a cup of Darjeeling tea and smell fresh jasmine flowers, I close my eyes and meditate; often, I can smell that beautiful fragrance.

In memory of Pondichéry I have created a fragrance that's reminiscent of Goa. I have named it Cafuné, which in Portuguese means 'tenderly running your fingers through your lover's hair'. The words 'I must go down to the seas again' often echo in my heart when it is weighed down by the heaviness of city life. This blend of lavender, frangipani, lemongrass and bergamot addresses my yearning for the wind and the whiff of salt spray, and transports me to the emerald waters in just a spritz.

A WHIFF OF MEMORY

My tryst with Cacharel's Anais Anais goes back to the time I encountered Dior's Poison. From the same trip in 1986, my mother had brought back this delicate little fragrance for my sister and me (yes, in those days, siblings shared such things). The pearly-white bottle with a pastel pink flower won my heart and became my symbol for all things feminine. The first sniff of it transported me to a dreamworld where everything was soft, fragile, delicate and floral. What I love about this perfume is that it does not fade away as most light fragrances do. This is because the base of the fragrance has sandalwood, vetiver, amber, cedarwood and oak moss.

The notes of tuberose, sandalwood and vetiver give this fragrance a touch of Indian summer and make it perfect for chiffons, pearls and all things feminine. This perfume reminds me of my aunt, who was married into the royal Khan family of Narajol, West Bengal, and had elaborate beauty rituals that sounded like the stuff of dreams. For instance, she would have her hair dried with fumes from a *dhunachi* (an incense burner) to ward off negativity and fragrance the room. My memory of her is a vision of white (I have always seen her wearing a simple white saree, yet looking gorgeous as ever). Her complexion was pink and the only adornment she wore was a whiff of something floral around her. I don't know what perfume she wore but her persona reminded me always of the pristine white bottle of Anais Anais. Inspired by the scent, I created the blend Saudade.

'Saudade' means 'nostalgia for a place or person far away'. This fragrance is also dedicated to my city of birth, Calcutta—a city that always somehow induces nostalgia for itself, its people, its culture, its food, its bygone days and more. The scent opens with a sparkle of neroli, leads to the amorous heart of jasmine and leaves a trail of sandalwood and myrrh.

LEGEND IN A BOTTLE

Think perfume and it is next to impossible not to come up with Chanel No. 5. It is obvious, natural and almost instinctive to do so. And why not? Generations of women have grown up wearing it (and swearing by it). Since its debut in 1921 the fragrance has been the sophisticate's choice and yet, to date, it remains an enigma—a quality that is underscored by its compelling commercials that end with the words 'Chanel No. 5' whispered in the background. These three words conjure up a sense of mystery and a desire to reach out for that classic magic potion.

A simple, straight-lined bottle and an equally unassuming name—what magic does this potion hold? Its heady vapours prompted Marilyn Monroe to famously claim that she wore only Chanel No. 5 to bed. Its loyalists swear that the fragrance is indeed an enigma, and the brand declares that 'trying to seize the magic of this strange osmosis is a pointless effort. Because fragrance, like love, has reasons that surpass reason'. Perhaps that's the stuff legends are made of, and you need to experience it yourself to be part of that magic.

But experiencing Chanel No. 5 is not just about wearing it. It involves knowing the history of the brand, understanding its unique composition and wearing it in style. From the very beginning the fragrance has been a symbol of mystery and allure, and over the decades the image of the perfume became seductive and sacred.

In a way, the perfume's fate was made the day Mademoiselle Chanel instructed the famous perfumer Ernest Beaux to create 'a women's fragrance that smells like women'. So at the heart of the composition lay a message that would empower women. The legend goes that Beaux presented Mlle Chanel with several options; and she chose the fifth sample, and thus the name Chanel No. 5.

Interestingly, the first spokesperson of the perfume was none other than Coco Chanel herself. She modelled for only one advertisement and that was for Chanel No. 5; its print advertisement first appeared in *Harper's Bazaar* in 1937. Since then, iconic beauties such as Marilyn Monroe, Catherine Deneuve, Carole Bouquet, Estella Warren, Nicole Kidman and Audrey Tautou have represented this fragrance. And each of them has contributed to the fantasy with her own charm and style.

For me, the one person—the one moment, the one picture—that crystallizes the enigma of this perfume is the photograph of Marilyn Monroe splashing our Chanel No 5. It is supposedly a candid shot that was taken just before the first performance of the play *Cat on a Hot Tin Roof*. A print of this iconic picture hangs on my studio wall, inspiring me to be who I am meant to be.

I have attempted an interpretation of this legendary fragrance. Here, I would like to underscore that all my inspired blends are merely my interpretations of these fragrances. So my ode to Chanel No. 5 is a blend of sandalwood, vanilla, jasmine, desi gulab and lavender.

GARDEN OF LOVE

When speaking of legendary perfumes and floral scents that have inspired me, I must remember the iconic Guerlain's Shalimar. There's so much already been spoken and written about this celebrated scent that it may seem that there is not much to add to it. However, that is perhaps the mystique of this fragrance. Even after almost a century after it was created, this blend is open to interpretation.

Shalimar was created by Jacques Guerlain, who was inspired by the eternal love story of the Mughal Emperor Shah Jahan and his consort Mumtaz Mahal. Apart from the Taj Mahal, Shah Jahan had created the Shalimar Bagh in Lahore in honour of his queen. This beautiful garden had also served as an inspiration for the Shalimar perfume. It is indeed an intriguing scent with notes of bergamot, rose, iris, jasmine, vanilla and tonka beans.

However, I must admit that, while I like the composition and complexity of the scent, it is a bit overpowering. So I tried creating something that would be similar in spirit. For inspiration, I turned to Kashmir, specifically to Srinagar and River Jhelum. Incidentally, there's the famous Shalimar Bagh (Shalimar is a Sanskrit word meaning 'temple of love') in Srinagar, which was built by none other than Emperor Jehangir and, of course, was dedicated to his queen Mehrunisa.

I have already spoken about the love story of this royal couple. There is something about their lives and romance that keeps drawing me to them. As an ode to their eternal love and Kashmir, and as an interpretation of the scent Shalimar,

I have created my fragrance blend Fanaa. The word 'Fanaa' means the 'annihilation' (as in Sufism) of the individual human will before the will of God. The keynote of this blend is blue lotus essential oil, which is sensuous and seductive. It is complemented with the accents of lavender, rosewood, saffron and cardamom.

SCENT OF PARADISE

In the winter of 2013, while Delhi was still reeling under the chill of a severe cold wave, I headed to the exotic locales of Koh Samui, Thailand, for the launch of Bulgari Omnia Coral. The caressing sun, breeze and sea, and the lazy afternoon, slowly and silently rolling into balmy evenings, lulled me into believing that spring was forever, and worked as a perfect setting for the launch of this fruity floral perfume.

The Bulgari Omnia collection is a range that's inspired by gemstones. In keeping with this tradition, it was a delicate coral necklace from the house of Bulgari that spurred the creation of Omnia Coral. The fresh youthful fragrance was symbolic of the coral and was like a whiff of good health— which is what coral promotes. Omnia Coral is one of the most beautiful compositions of fruity floral notes I have ever encountered. The first whiff of the scent greets you with a burst of citrusy bergamot and goji berries, then leads you into the juicy notes of pomegranate and hibiscus, and finally envelopes you in the warm, sensuous fumes of musk.

The perfume is a heady mix and is just perfect for a romantic summer evening. This scent appeals to the Bengali in me. I guess it has a lot to do with the coral—something that married Bengali women wear—and the hibiscus flower, which is offered to Goddess Kali. I see it as a fragrance infused with intense, earthy energy.

I have worn this perfume with a white shift dress and delicate coral jewellery. However, I love wearing it with red and white sarees—not just the Bengal Taant sarees but sarees in that combination. I keep make-up minimal, with a hint of peachy-coral tint on the lips and sheer gloss mascara on the lashes. I pull the hair back in a neat bun and tuck in a vibrant hibiscus.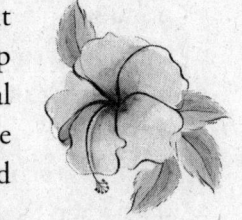

Inspired by the vivaciousness of this fragrance I have created a fruity floral with essential oils and Bach flower remedies: In a 10 ml bottle I put in 4 drops each of sandalwood, vetiver, cedarwood and pine; followed by 4 drops of lavender; 2 drops each of mogra, rajnigandha and desi gulab; and 1 drop each of ylang-ylang and neroli. To this I add 2 drops each of lemon and bergamot. The rest of the bottle I top up with honeysuckle Bach flower remedy. I allow the mix to rest for forty-eight hours before using it.

BED OF ROSES

In my stint at *Harper's Bazaar*, India, as beauty editor, I taught myself to understand and appreciate the narrative of a perfume. When you adopt the fable, the fragrance also starts adapting to your style and sensibilities.

For instance, in 2011, when Burberry Body perfume was launched, I got a chance to interview Christopher Bailey, who was then the chief creative officer of the brand. It was the sheer excitement of that conversation that made me fall in love with the fragrance, and to date it remains my favourite daywear perfume.

Just a couple of hours before my scheduled interview I had received a small, unassuming bottle with an equally nondescript label—it was a sample (not an actual bottle, but a preview of sorts) of the perfume, Burberry Body. Though the press kit with the images and perfume details had prepared me for a very special fragrance, it was only after the first burst of fresh peach and mysterious absinthe vapours that I realized that what I had in hand was not just another scent of the season. It was a fragrance that was here to stay.

What won my heart were the heart notes of rose and the trail of sandalwood. Burberry Body is undoubtedly very British, yet it is a fragrance that can be perfect for any time and place. During the interview, Bailey said that this perfume was inspired by the trench coat, which has seen so many adaptations and interpretations. I find the trench coat very difficult to accept as a versatile garment but the perfume is indeed flexible, adaptable . . . adoptable. Inspired by this rosy fragrance, I created my perfume blend called Rooh. It is a concentrate of vetiver, cedarwood and desi gulab. I like to describe it as the scent of my soul.

AN ENIGMA

From *Harper's Bazaar*, I moved into a marketing role at Sephora India. Every time I visited the store, I would take time out to smell about 3–4 fragrances. One day, Tom Ford's Black Orchid bottles arrived at the store and when I spritzed on a little of the perfume, its first burst of spicy intoxicating notes hit my head. However, soon it mellowed into something floral, velvety and sexy. There is something about this fragrance that makes it mysterious and unfathomable. The best part is it lasts on my skin, like forever—which is a very rare thing for a modern perfume to have achieved.

This perfume is an out-and-out noir fragrance, and you should completely avoid it during the day, unless it is an extremely cold day or you are feeling vulnerable. In fact, you should wear it to feel empowered. I love wearing it with silk sarees or anything sexy in black or shades of wine.

My perfume blend Flambé can be considered as an ode to Tom Ford's Black Orchid. Flambe definitely doesn't smell like Black Orchid but its spirit is akin to that of Black Orchid's.

Like Black Orchid, Flambé has spicy, sweet and floral notes, and is as flamboyant as it can get. It is a blend of vanilla, oud, rose, black pepper and tangerine. Black pepper and tangerine create a bold, heady introduction to the fragrance. The note of rose keeps the heart of the scent peppery, velvety and intense. Vanilla and oud help the fragrance to linger longer with a sweet, woody trail.

LEAVING A TRAIL

When speaking of scents, it would remain incomplete if we didn't talk about the art of wearing fragrances. Of course, there are the popular tips like wearing the scent on pulse points, or spraying a cloud of perfume before you and then stepping into that fume, finding that 'one' signature scent, and so on. However, my dabbling with perfumery has changed my views on perfume wearing.

Of late, I have been breaking rules. Mixing scents was considered to be almost blasphemous. But I am enjoying doing just that. This season I am enjoying mixing four types of fragrances. I am using pure geranium oil on my pulse points and Tom Ford's Black Orchid as my base, followed by Ajmal Perfumes' Amber Magic, and I finish with a flourish of my own Jhelum Loves' Flambé.

I am also experimenting with wearing different perfumes on different parts of the body. I like wearing something earthy with notes of vetiver or patchouli behind my knees, woody florals on the stomach and lower back, spicy floral notes on the chest, citrusy notes of neroli or bergamot around the neck, and heady notes of lotus, oud, jasmine or sandalwood on the hair.

In both ways that I am experimenting perfume wearing, there is one thing I focus on and that is what I call my signature. So my 'signature' are floral notes, as I feel that the scent of flowers offers the most versatile and dynamic platform for perfume-building. Keeping this in mind, I try to weave in other fragrances.

So what happens when you start dabbling with scents and soak them into your very being? It definitely sharpens your senses and you become more aware of yourself and surroundings. As for me, I get asked very interesting questions. At a recent event someone asked me, 'Do you think spirits can communicate through scents?'

I smiled and quoted Rumi. 'Love bears the fragrance of musk. What choice does it have but to spread and be recognized?'

PART 4

ADORNMENTS & ANOINTMENTS

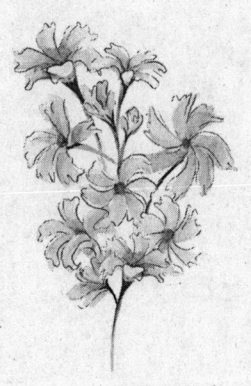

FLORAL EMBRACE

In school, summer vacations meant either a trip to some hill station or cousins visiting us. However, during one summer break we went to visit my mother's grandmother in Midnapore, a small town near Calcutta. I was not very happy about this, because I was always a little intimidated by my great-grandmother. She always looked stern and formidable. I don't remember much of her, and I certainly can't think of remembering her ever smile.

She was a stickler for rules and everything had to run by the clock as per routine. I hated it. But one afternoon, she took me to visit some distant cousin of ours. After all these years, I can't even remember that cousin's face or name, but what I do remember is her showing me how to make flower ornaments for ourselves and for our dolls, because it was a doll's wedding, she had explained.

Now, this was something that I had never seen before. At home, in Calcutta, we had a huge cabinet full of dolls. It was like a mini museum my mother had painstakingly curated; and playing with those dolls was strictly forbidden.

I had other dolls—the ones with those ghostly blue eyes and straw-like blonde hair. But on rare occasions the dolls in the showcase were brought out, and I could play with them for a while, under my mother's supervision.

But no such rules applied to this cousin of mine. She reverentially adorned the dolls with delicate floral ornaments that looked so pristine and fragrant. It reminded me of the way one of my aunts would take care of her Radha and Krishna idols at the temple in her house. Till then, I knew flowers to be offered only to gods and goddesses in religious ceremonies, or in weddings as garlands. So when I saw dolls being dressed in blooms, my perception of dolls and idols merged.

'Who Let The Dolls Out?'

Her days were with them.
At night she fed, bathed and put them to bed.
Generations passed . . .
I wished my days could also be with them.
Rather than looking through the glass wall,
I wished I could take them to bed.

But rules were rules.
Locked in temples and cabinets,
our loves must remain.
She was ordered to care,
I was allowed to see.
She couldn't step out,
I could never step in.

She longed to seek them
beyond the boundary walls,
just crossing that line, into that field.

I sought to enter that glass globe,
waiting with bated breath for the clock to strike,
the gossamer fabric of time to split,
so I could slip in,
falling into that magical world of light and glitter.
Just there, but just a little further.

And it happened one day . . .
She didn't ring the bell,
I didn't seek the permission.
The lines were crossed.

Who let the dolls out?
It was she, it was me.
Was it me? Was it she?
She walked out carrying him,
seeking him.
I sneaked her out,
locked her in, in a trunk,
so no big hunk could steal her away from me.

We wandered, we wondered,
we sought, we were sought.
Fleetingly we saw ourselves,
when our paths crossed.

Did she find him?
Did I release her?
Did she release him?
Did I find her?

She called them Radha–Krishna.
Years went by, images changed.
glass was fragile, wax would melt.
Clay was cheap, porcelain beyond reach.
So plastic they had to be to recast as Barbie and Ken.

The cacophony rises again.
'Come come, Barbie, let's go party', 'Radha likes to
party', dolls are idols;
idols are dolls.
The poet becomes the prophet,
the prophet becomes the puppet.
It's time to churn, break, melt and remould them all.

Bubble, bubble, toil and trouble,
I shiver, I shake, I rage, I crumble.
Will I break what I create . . .
I cast off the transient,
but will the truth unveil?

FLORAL WEDDING JEWELLERY

Flowers have long been part of a woman's adornments
in Indian customs. In fact, in the traditional concept of
'Sola Shringar' (sixteen adornments), wearing flowers was
considered an integral part of a woman's grooming ritual. In
fact, Sola Shringar is not just adornments; it is an art, a skill
that women were expected to master. It also included the art
of preparing and eating paan.

More recently, Anushka Sharma, Deepika Padukone and Priyanka Chopra made this tradition a raging trend by decking up in flowers for their mehendi ceremony. With *kaanphool* (floral jewellery for the ears) to *hathphool* (floral jewellery that is worn on hands starting from the finger and clasping the wrists), from anklets to gorgeous veils—the trend of wearing flower jewellery is here to stay. Its popularity is such that it has inspired a dish mentioned in the chapter 'Food & Flavours' of this book.

In traditional Bengali weddings the bride wears floral jewellery during the haldi ceremony in the morning of the wedding day, and on the reception day, the bride and nuptial bed (it is, in fact, called the *phool shojja* or 'bed of flowers') is bedecked with flowers like rajnigandha, mogra and gulab. Almost always it is a combination of red and white blooms—a colour-pairing that symbolizes purity and passion. These three flowers—gulab, mogra and rajnigandha—have fragrant notes that are at once calming and aphrodisiacal. In some ways, the nuptial room can be seen as an amorous aromatherapy chamber.

FLORAL MOTIFS IN JEWELLERY

While fresh flowers have been fashioned as ornaments, fashion jewellery has in turn drawn inspiration from blooms. And to understand it better I had a chat with the founders of jewellery brand Zariin Jewelry—Mamta and Vidhi Gupta. I fondly refer to them as the Zariin girls. Two of their recent collections have been inspired by flowers—Gold Blooms and Florets. What intrigued them the most while creating this line is the fact that nothing in nature, including flowers, follows a set rule or pattern; yet there is an alignment. The duo's greatest satisfaction is being able to capture the delicate structure of the petals in a material as powerful as metal.

In terms of traditional jewellery, they tell me that flowers like lotus, rose, jasmine and marigold not only make a significant part of religious votives but also in jewellery motifs. A few distinctive examples are how the motifs were explored in three-dimensional forms in south Indian temple jewellery and in Meenakari jewellery that uses enamel techniques.

The sisters highlight the fact that the Mughal culture in the subcontinent introduced a combination of floral motifs with geometry. With Islam restricting the representation of human forms in artwork, these natural elements gained more significance.

Interestingly, gemstones of spectacular colours have been used to depict the colour array of flowers in jewellery—and this remains as relevant today. Taking me back to the history of jewellery, they explain that jewellery history can be closely associated with the art history of the place, which in turn is connected to the place's cultural history. India, being a rich melting point of distinctive cultures and religions, has an abundance of forms to take inspiration from, which is clearly visible in the sheer variety of craft and the floral patterns used in jewellery. Our handcrafted patterns set our jewellery apart from the otherwise prevalent industrial techniques.

I ask them for tips on wearing jewellery with floral motifs, and this is what they advise: 'Don't limit your florals to spring! The floral pattern is a classic, loved by all, and all year round. Contemporary aesthetics allow us to play with patterns—a fun approach of mix 'n' match. Use your floral jewellery to add that dose of nature to your outfit. It is a timeless trend and a versatile one that makes it so integral. Style it with your pants, suit, classic dress, casual denims or dreamy saree. Floral jewellery works with everything and one must make the most of this!'

FLOWERS IN FASHION

When I think of style involving flowers, fashion designer Nida Mahmood and the quintessential flower in her hair comes to mind. 'I think my personal style with flower corsages just happened,' she tells me. 'There was never any effort to create a statement.'

What else can it be? After all, few can carry off a flower with a short hair-crop and, particularly, the flower effortlessly pinned at one side of the forehead.

Flowers are an intrinsic part of Nida's work, quite naturally. In creating her designs, she draws inspiration from nature and India.

'I love the vintage Indian style of drawing flowers and have created many designs inspired by that style.'

I ask Nida if she has any favourite Indian flower. She does not; however, she says she loves the form of the lotus and the various ways in which it can be interpreted. And she has extensively used it in her designs over the years.

As we wrap up our chat, I ask her if she has any style tips to offer.

She says: 'Follow your style and let design speak to you. If a design speaks to you, it is for you.'

Speaking of flowers and fashion, I also caught up with fashion designer and yogini Malini Ramani. Her designs have a strong floral influence and her eclectic style quite naturally embraces blooms.

Malini loves styling herself with mogra garlands around her neck and wrists. The easiest way in which she lifts her mood is by tucking a champak flower behind her ear. Wearing a fresh bloom is indeed the best mood fix.

MAKE-UP MUSE

My favourite way of wearing flowers is actually wearing them. While I would love to wear a fresh bloom in my hair every day, I have to restrict myself to wearing floral clips, for practical purposes. I have a dozen of these in different shades and styles; and all I have to do is just clip them on to my hair.

I like to wear it behind the ear with my hair open or next to my messy bun. It is instant dress-up. Most of the days I gravitate towards red roses and I echo that in my make-up with a red lipstick (my all-time favourite is M.A.C lipstick in Ruby Woo). I sign off that look with kohl; I frame my eyes with a thick line of charcoal-black eye pencil or gel liner.

When I wear any flower, I try to incorporate its shade either in my eye make-up or lipstick. I have been lucky to work with several make-up artists to create flower-inspired looks. One of the most memorable ones was with Cory Walia, for *Harper's Bazaar India*'s first anniversary issue. We used four blooms as inspiration for four different looks. The most interesting one was the look with yellow eyeliner. Our inspiration was a Siddartha

Tytler dress with a striking yellow tulle flower on a shoulder. I remember Cory lining the upper lash with a bottle-green liner first and then using a bright yellow eyeshadow over the green liner. He had stretched the line out to give it a classic winged-liner look. For lip colour, he had used a shade of beige.

Make-up artist Anu Kaushik, with whom I have worked on several beauty shoots, is at her best when working with fresh flowers. She has created entire make-up looks with fresh blooms and petals. Speaking of flowers and make-up, Anu says, 'It's amazing that a mogra or marigold band on a simple braid instantly creates "Indian-ness", whereas roses in tied or open hair offer classic, vintage vibes. A sprinkle of baby's breath flowers in textured hair makes for a modern, easy look.' Lotus is Anu's favourite flower for make-up inspiration. Ranging from green, creamy white, pink and violet to deep berry, lotuses have a myriad of colours wrapped into each other. She incorporates these hues by using pastels and warm tones in eye make-up.

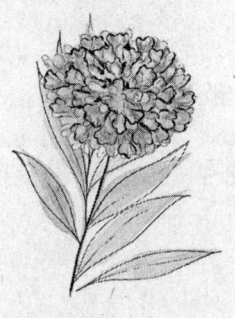

When it comes to bridal make-up, I am inclined (quite unapologetically) to say that my mother, Ruby Biswas, is one of the best. For the wedding day, she asks most of the brides to wear sarees in tones of red. This day's make-up is usually traditional and she dresses up the bride's hair with red and white flowers. However, for the reception day's make-up, she advises the brides to wear purples—blues, pinks or whatever colour they prefer.

For this look, I love to see her play with fresh flowers. In the morning she calls her florist and, with a tiny piece of the saree as her guide, she chooses fresh flowers that match exactly with the shade of the saree. After that, she instructs the florist to fashion those blooms into bands or garlands depending on the hairstyle she has in mind. Her favourite flowers for this look are gladioli, gerberas, carnations, scarlet and orange marigolds, roses and orchids.

She picks up eyeshadows reflecting the shades of the petals to do the eye make-up. She works with numerous eyeshadows in different hues and textures to create one look. Inglot eyeshadows and pigments are her favourites. For kohl and gel liner, she prefers Bobbi Brown or Clinique. When it comes to eye make-up, more is better for her. However, she teaches me that 'blending is the key; that's the test of a true make-up artist'. Hence, even if she has used 6–7 shades and forms of eye make-up, it all looks elegant. She often recommends brides to wear coloured contact lenses to highlight and complete the colour story.

Wish to create an easy flower-inspired look? Then try this simple yet gorgeous step-by-step party make-up by Chandni Singh.

Chandni uses the rustic, vibrant pink bougainvillea for inspiration and cues. 'I love bougainvillea, especially the pink variety, which is such a happy hue. It's dainty, sits well and looks particularly nice with Indian wear.' Follow the steps suggested by Chandni to create the look.

For Make-up

1. On clean skin, apply Jhelum Loves Bach Flower & Aroma Remedies Roseate Face Oil to hydrate skin.
2. Apply hydrating foundation and concealer where required.
3. Just set the under-eyes with little powder and gently dab powder on the skin with a powder brush so that it does not take away the glow.

4. Use M.A.C lipstick in Pink Pigeon on the eyelids and lips.
5. Dab on Benefit Benetint on lips and cheeks for the rosy glow.
6. Apply lots of mascara and with brown pencil fill in the brows to complete the look.
7. Seal the look with GlamGlow Glowsetter Makeup Setting Mist.

For Hairstyling

1. Make a ponytail with your hair at the height where you want your bun.
2. Once done, pinch some hair out on the crown and front section with your fingers to create texture.
3. Use a hair donut and let it go through your ponytail.
4. Now take hair sections, tease them a bit and cover entire area of the hair donut.
5. Secure with thin bobby pins to create a bun.
6. Fix bougainvillea flowers all around the bun or on one side, as you like it.
7. Spray on a shine spray like BBlunt Mini Spotlight Hair Polish for Instant Shine.

HEALING BLOOMS

In a paper titled 'Introduction to Pushpa Ayurveda',* author K.P. Vardhan describes how flower therapy or Pushpa Ayurveda was developed as a branch of Ayurveda. Prior to the development of Pushpa Ayurveda, traditional Ayurveda had used animal and bird by-products for healing. Vardhan

---

* K.P. Vardhan, 'Introduction to Pushpa Ayurveda', *Ancient Science of Life*, vol. iv, no. 3, January 1985, pp. 153–57.

claims that it was Vardhamana Mahavira's belief in ahimsa that inspired the discovery of treatments with flowers.

According to Pushpa Ayurveda, flowers can be used for healing in five sensorial ways: seeing, adorning, anointing, smelling and consuming. The chapters 'Essence & Emotions' and 'Scents & Sensuality' have addressed the last two healing aspects. What I wish to focus here is on adornments and anointments. Both these facets of healing focus on the sense of touch. In ancient times, a patient would be advised to *wear* flowers as garments and ornaments, or would be made to lie down on a bed of flowers. How beautiful is that! This goes to show that, perhaps, the concept of wearing floral ornaments during weddings has roots in this ancient healing practice. What was once such a gorgeous healing technique, I guess, has been reduced, due to ravages of time, to just a ritual on a special day.

BLOOM SERVICE

The other tactile healing with flowers was through anointments, a method in which flowers alone or mixed with some other healing herb was made into a paste and applied on the patient. This application of floral packs has survived in modern times through DIY and spa rituals involving scrubs, packs and wraps.

FLORAL ANOINTMENT

Combining my practices of Bach flower remedies, aromatherapy, yoga and meditation, I have developed my own method of chakra healing. For this therapy, I have developed seven blends of essential oils and flower essences, wherein each blend is used to anoint and activate a corresponding chakra. There are seven main chakras: *mooladhar*/root, *swadishthan*/sacral, *manipura*/solar plexus, *anahata*/heart, *vishudhi*/throat, *ajna*/third eye and *sahasrara*/ crown. My aromatherapy guru, Dr Ravi Ratan, opines that essential oils can be categorized into seven different groups based on the chakras they influence. Dr Ratan believes that different parts of a plant correspond to different chakras and, therefore, their essential oils likewise resonate with different chakras.

So for instance, root oils like vetiver and patchouli affect the root chakra; the bark oils sandalwood and cedarwood affect the sacral chakra; spice oils like cinnamon, clove and black pepper resonate with the solar plexus; flower oils like rose, jasmine and geranium activate the heart chakra; fruit oils like lemon, orange, mandarin and bergamot affect the throat chakra; and leaf oils like mint, holy basil, bail and clary sage resonate with the third eye chakra and are linked to spirituality. Sandalwood, frangipani, blue lotus, jatamansi and immortelle essential oils open up the crown chakra.

However, I feel that chakras can be activated with a specific flower oil, and a specific flower essence has attributes which synergize with a particular chakra.

SO WHAT ARE CHAKRAS?

Simply, they are energy vortexes. However, there is much more to it. What is especially relevant to this book is that each chakra is represented by a lotus flower.

ACTIVATING CHAKRAS

To cleanse, energize and balance each chakra, understand each chakra and the way to anoint them—to bring out their best.

FIRST CHAKRA

We begin at the first chakra,
located at the base of your spine.
The mooladhar, or root chakra, is red.
It includes the feet and legs.
Its teachings come from your tribe,
or family of origin.
It's how you walk on the earth,
integrating the lessons you've learned
with the beliefs you've formed.

Symbol: Four-petalled lotus flower.
Anointment: Anoint the root chakra with Jhelum Loves Balance Chakra Oil by applying it on the area, once anticlockwise and thrice clockwise.
Flower oil: Geranium essential oil balances hormones and is excellent for skin and hair care.
Flower essence: Clematis Bach flower remedy roots you to the present, and is ideal for activating the root chakra.
Benefits: Promotes grounding and increases vitality.

SECOND CHAKRA

The second chakra is seated
two fingers below your navel.

The swadishthan or sacral chakra is orange.
It's weighed down by
hurt, anger, rejection, lust and greed.
When balanced, it helps savour life,
with all its flavour and creativity.

Symbol: Six-petalled lotus flower.
Anointment: Anoint the sacral chakra with Jhelum Loves Passion Chakra Oil by applying it on the area, once anticlockwise and thrice clockwise.
Flower oil: Jasmine essential oil is calming and aphrodisiacal.
Flower essence: Cherry plum helps control outbursts.
Benefits: Improves circulation and helps balance emotions.

THIRD CHAKRA

The third chakra is located
at the solar plexus,
positioned and whirling
between the navel and diaphragm.
Manipura or solar plexus chakra is yellow.
This represents who you are,
one on one to the world.
It empowers your self-esteem and personality.
You'll feel it there energetically,
when your passions create your destiny.

Symbol: Ten-petalled lotus flower.
Anointment: Anoint the solar plexus chakra with Jhelum Loves Strength Chakra Oil by applying it on the area, once anticlockwise and thrice clockwise.

Flower oil: Ylang-ylang essential oil has anti-inflammatory properties and is ideal for the solar plexus chakra.

Flower essence: Vervain Bach flower remedy helps channelize the fire energy.

Benefits: Improves digestion and strengthens willpower.

FOURTH CHAKRA

The fourth chakra is nestled
at the centre of the chest.
The anahata, or heart chakra, is green.
It governs compassion for the self and others;
heals and nurtures a broken heart,
smothered dreams and rejected love.
Tap on it ever so gently
to love yourself and others unconditionally.

Symbol: Twelve-petalled lotus flower.

Anointment: Anoint the heart chakra with Jhelum Loves Love Chakra Oil by applying it on the area, once anticlockwise and thrice clockwise.

Flower oil: Rose essential oil without a doubt is the oil for the heart chakra. It promotes love, compassion, courage and healing.

Flower essence: Holly Bach flower remedy helps dissolve jealousy and makes way for divine love to flow through.

Benefits: Strengthens heart and lungs. Promotes courage, compassion and forgiveness.

FIFTH CHAKRA

The fifth chakra is located
at the base of the throat.
The vishuddhi, or throat chakra, is blue.
It helps in correct communication,
expressing emotions and opinions with clarity.
Activate it with chants and songs,
and see how it fills your life
with flowing rhythm and sweet symphony.

Symbol: Sixteen-petalled lotus flower.
Anointment: Anoint the throat chakra, located under the navel, with Jhelum Loves Express Chakra Oil, by applying it on the area once anticlockwise and thrice clockwise.
Flower oil: Neroli is a beautiful essential oil that brings instant cheer.
Flower essence: Centaury Bach flower remedy helps in expressing one's thoughts and emotions correctly.
Benefits: Cures throat ailments; helps in self-expression.

SIXTH CHAKRA

The sixth chakra is present
just between the brows.
The ajna, or third-eye chakra, is indigo.
It houses telepathy and instincts.
It sharpens perception and awakens intuition.
If you meditate on it,
your subconscious mind is revealed.
Your pair of physical eyes observes
the theatrics of the outside world.

But the third-eye looks inward,
directing the movie of your life and the universe.

Symbol: Two-petalled lotus flower.
Anointment: Anoint the third-eye chakra with Jhelum Loves Intuition Chakra Oil, by applying it on the area once anticlockwise and thrice clockwise.
Flower oil: The only essential oil that comes to my mind is the blue lotus. This oil is aphrodisiacal, but it is also excellent for meditation.
Flower essence: Wild oat Bach flower remedy, which helps one get a direction in life.
Benefits: Helps achieve clarity and improves intuition.

SEVENTH CHAKRA

The seventh chakra is situated
at the crown of your head.
The sahasrara, or crown chakra, can be either pink, white or violet.
This is the connection to the universe;
when activated with self-transformation,
your life pulsates with divine love and wisdom.

Symbol: 100-petalled lotus flower.
Anointment: Anoint the crown chakra with Jhelum Loves Passion Chakra Oil, by applying it on the area once anticlockwise and thrice clockwise.
Flower oil: Frangipani essential oil has regenerative properties.
Flower essence: White chestnut Bach flower remedy—it gets rid of unnecessary mental chatter and helps one be mindful of the present.
Benefits: Helps achieve clarity and wisdom.

Every day, spend a few moments
meditating on your chakras
by focusing on your breath,
and symbolic lotus flowers or rainbow colours.
Observe your body and mind,
make note of issues that bother.
Then spin the chakras one by one
by applying the floral blends
on their corresponding chakra points,
first anticlockwise,
and then clockwise.
Take a deep breath in,
sing the sargam thrice.
Transform the negativity,
breathe out the excess energy.
Seek blessings of the universe;
bless the earth and ground that you stand on.

PASTES, PACKS AND PASSIONS

When I stir up beauty recipes, I am in my element. I so love what I do that I often say, 'I do what I dream; I dream what I do.' And I pray to the universe that this may remain forever true.

My studio and kitchen are often hit by these frenzied moments of creativity, when I bring out on my worktable bottles of oils, essences, fresh flowers and whatever else my mind fancies. These are moments when the spirit of the flower witch within me gets its full expression. I am in the throes of passion by accident: Just a smell, word, memory, taste, sight, touch, song, mood—anything sensorial or emotional can trigger this happy madness. And with immediate effect that recipe/innovation/creation has to be instantly manifested.

I am lucky that I am surrounded by very gentle, generous and extremely patient souls who are forever ready for experiments.

CATCH 55

Some of the recipes below are results of my moments of madness, which I have sometimes created on my own, at times with my mother, Ruby Biswas, and my colleague, Shruti Anand. The others have been generously shared by my friends Kshama Shamsukha, Aparna Gupta and Vasudha Rai; Ayurveds Dr Ipsita Chatterjee and Dr Sharad Kulkarni; and by beauty brands like RAS Luxury Oils.

CRAB APPLE

This is a Bach flower remedy that helps in cleansing. In combination with Rescue Remedy (an emergency fix made of five other Bach flower remedies—impatiens, star of Bethlehem, rock rose, clematis and cherry plum, and crab apple), it is excellent for hair and skin care. Just add a few drops of crab apple in any face wash, shampoo, soap, toner, oil, cream or pack to heal and rejuvenate your hair and skin.

While, of course, you can add this to all the recipes to follow, here are some of the simplest ways in which you can incorporate this versatile flower essence in your regimen.

- **Crab apple and coconut oil cleanser:** In pure, cold-pressed coconut oil (1 tsp) add crab apple Bach flower remedy (4–6 drops). Use this to remove your make-up as well as moisturize your skin.

With your fingertips, apply the oil over your eyes and lips. Leave it for a few seconds and then wipe it off with a soft wet tissue. Splash your face with water to remove residue. Pat dry and apply the remaining oil mix as a moisturizer on your face. You can use the same mix to condition your strands and scalp before a hair wash.

- **Crab apple and tea tree mist:** Fill a 60 ml spray bottle with mineral water. Add in tea tree essential oil (2 drops), crab apple Bach flower remedy (8 drops) and Rescue Remedy (4 drops). This is a great spray that fights acne and dandruff.
- **Crab apple and aloe vera gel mask:** In aloe vera gel (1 tbsp) add crab apple and white chestnut Bach flower remedies (4–5 drops each) and fresh turmeric paste (¼ tsp). Apply this on a clean face and leave it on for twenty minutes. Wash off with lukewarm water. This gives your face a golden glow and is suitable for all skin types.

HONEY

Of course, it is not a flower but is one of the best by-products of blooms. Honey is antibacterial, a rich antioxidant, an excellent cleanser and moisturizer. Therefore, it can be used to fight acne, condition the skin and fight premature signs of ageing. It also reduces hair fall, fights dandruff and cleans the scalp.

- **Honey and lemon cleanser:** For dull skin, add lemon zest (½ tsp) in honey (1 tsp) and a few drops of lemon juice. Mix it together and apply it on your face. Massage the face with this cleanser for five minutes and wash off with lukewarm water. Skin will look bright and feel soft.
- **Honey and egg face pack:** If you have oily skin, whisk together honey (1 tbsp) and egg white (1) and apply the mix on your face. Leave it for twenty minutes to dry. Wash off with cold water. For normal to dry skin, use the yolk instead of the egg white and follow the same procedure. You may add a drop each of tea tree and lemon essential oils if you wish. This pack helps tighten and brighten skin.
- **Honey and fresh cream face pack:** To invigorate dry and mature skin, mix together honey (1 tsp) and fresh cream (1 tsp) and apply it on your face and neck. Leave it on for ten minutes and then gently massage it for two to three minutes. Wash off with warm water.
- **Honey and olive oil hair treatment:** To promote hair growth and scalp health, warm olive oil (1 tbsp) and add to it honey (2 tsp) and fresh ginger juice (¼ tsp). Mix well and massage on to the scalp, and spread it along the hair strand. Leave it for twenty minutes and shampoo as usual.
- **Honey and banana hair mask:** To bring life and bounce into your hair, mash two ripe bananas and mix with 1 tbsp of honey and apply it on your hair and scalp. Cover the head with a shower cap and

leave it on for twenty minutes. Rinse off the pack and then shampoo.

- **Honey and oatmeal body scrub**: To exfoliate and invigorate your skin, mix together honey (1 tbsp), oatmeal (1 tbsp), sweet almond oil (1 tbsp) and coffee powder (1 tbsp) and massage it on to face and body. Add a drop of vanilla extract to the scrub to make it smell more delicious. This is optional. Wash off after fifteen minutes.

- **Honey and papaya anti-ageing face mask**: For firm, youthful skin, mix together honey (1 tbsp), mashed ripe papaya (1 tbsp) and dahi (1 tbsp). Apply the mixture on your face and leave it on for thirty minutes. You can also massage the mixture as you apply it, as doing so improves blood circulation and tightens the skin. Wash off with warm water.

- **Honey, sugar and cinnamon lip scrub**: To exfoliate and plump lips, use a scrub made of honey (1 tsp), sugar (1 tsp), lemon juice (1 tsp) and cinnamon powder (1 tsp). Massage for two minutes and leave it on for five minutes. Wipe off with water.

CLOVE

This spice is a dried bud and has been used for ages for its antibacterial properties. It is also rich in antioxidants. Dr Chatterjee explains that in Ayurvedic texts, clove bud is referred to as *sriprasun*, which means the flower of gods, and *chandanpushpak*, meaning 'with fragrance of sandalwood'. Most beauty recipes use clove essential oil. The DIY treatments below use clove essential oil, clove bud powder and whole clove buds.

- **Clove oil and aloe vera juice toner:** Clove bud oil is excellent for treating acne but should never be used directly on skin. Dr Chatterjee says, 'Make a toner with aloe vera juice and then apply.' Fill a 60 ml spray bottle with aloe vera juice and add 2 drops of clove bud essential oil in it. Shake it well and spray it on the area affected by acne. Store it in the refrigerator.
- **Clove-infused coconut hair oil:** To treat dandruff and improve blood circulation in the scalp, warm coconut oil (1 tbsp) with freshly dry-roasted clove buds (4–5). Strain out the clove buds and massage the oil into the scalp. Leave for twenty minutes and then shampoo as usual.
- **Clove bud and orange body scrub:** For exfoliating and revitalizing your skin, mix together clove bud powder (1 tbsp), orange peel powder (1 tbsp), finely ground sugar (1 tbsp) and milk powder (1 tbsp) with orange juice (2 tbsp) to create a paste, and massage that on to your face and body for five to ten minutes. Wash off with lukewarm water.
- **Clove bud and cypress oil deodorant:** To keep your feet and armpits smelling fresh, mix together clove bud powder (1 tsp), cypress essential oil (4 drops), baking powder (1 tbsp) and olive oil (1 tbsp), and apply the paste on your armpits and feet. Leave it for ten minutes and wash off.

SAFFRON

Like clove, saffron or kesar is a flower and it is as beneficial for skin as it is richly fragrant in meals. This spice is rich in vitamins and has anti-inflammatory properties, which makes it a perfect ingredient for treating acne and sensitive skin.

- **Kesar, turmeric and milk face pack:** For healthy glowing skin, warm milk (1 tbsp) and dissolve in it milk powder (1 tsp), grated fresh turmeric (½ tsp), cornflour (¼ tsp) and saffron (4–5 strands). Simmer the mixture on low flame till it forms a thick golden yellow paste. Cool it and apply it on face and neck. Leave it on for twenty minutes and wash off with lukewarm water.

- **Kesar and almond face cleanser:** This paste will draw out dirt from your skin pores better than any charcoal pack—that's my conviction. Pound together 3–4 almonds (soaked overnight in milk or water) and 4–5 strands of saffron. Make a paste with this powder and milk or plain water (1 tsp). Apply the paste on your face and neck and let it dry. Take a few drops of water and gently massage the skin till the paste comes off along with dirt and dead skin.

- **Kesar and papaya enzyme peel:** Mash ripe papaya (2 tsp) with saffron (4–5 strands). Apply this on clean face and neck and leave it on for fifteen minutes. Wipe it off with a cotton ball dipped in raw milk. This ritual is excellent for dry, mature skin.

- **Kesar, turmeric and chickpea flour pack:** For dry skin, blend together saffron strands (4–5), chickpea flour (1 tsp), grated fresh turmeric (¼ tsp) and cold milk (1 tsp). You can cut open a vitamin E capsule and add its contents to this pack. Apply on face and neck and allow it to dry for twenty minutes. Gently massage with a little cold water to remove the pack. Wash off with water. It stimulates the skin and leaves it soft and glowing. For oily skin, use lemon juice in place of milk.

ROSE

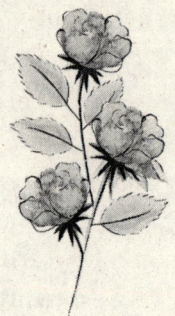

This flower, I think, is the most popular flower in beauty care and I am especially fond of the desi gulab. Rose heals emotions and is excellent for skin and hair care. It is cleansing, calming, moisturizing and promotes youthfulness.

- **Desi gulab and green tea ice pack**: To remove under-eye dark circles, take a cup of green tea liquor and mix with it almond oil (¼ tsp) and crushed desi gulab petals (½ tsp). Freeze this in an ice tray. Once a day, take one ice cube in a soft cotton cloth or gauze and gently press it around your eyes for three to five minutes.

(by Ruby Biswas)

- **Desi gulab and jojoba oil lip scrub**: Grind together fresh desi gulab petals (2 tsp), jojoba oil (2 tsp) with almonds (4–5) soaked overnight in milk. This makes a sweet-smelling lip scrub that exfoliates and instantly moisturizes your lips.

(by Ruby Biswas)

- **Desi gulab and dal body scrub**: Grind together masoor dal (2 tbsp) and moong dal (2 tbsp), and then add crushed, dry desi gulab petals (2 tbsp) to it. Store it, and before bath, take a fistful of the mix and add little milk to it to make a thick paste. Apply this pack over body and massage gently for ten minutes and wash off.

(by Sheela Anand)

- **Desi gulab and milk bath**: Mix together baking powder (4 tbsp), milk (4 tbsp), cornflour (4 tbsp) and dried and crushed desi gulab petals (4 tbsp). Either you can add this mix to your bath water or you can scrub your face and body with the paste mix and wash off after fifteen minutes.

- **Desi gulab and sandalwood face pack**: As a child the first religious duty that was assigned to me during any puja in the house was to make sandalwood paste. On a traditional flat, round stone grinder, I used to put a few drops of water and, with a thick sandalwood piece, rub the stone to make sandalwood paste. I loved doing this chore because it fascinated me how a fragrant paste could be made with a piece of stone and wood. Now, I have this contraption at home and I often make sandalwood paste for home-grown beauty treatments. One of my favourites is this pack:

    On the stone slab, grind together poppy seeds (½ tsp), dried rose petals (1 tsp) and raw milk (1 tsp) with the sandalwood stick. Keep grinding it all together till it makes a fine paste. Apply the paste on face and leave it on for twenty minutes. Wash off with water. This is a great face pack for summer and is effective for all skin types.

- **Desi gulab and rice flour scrub**: To remove tan, make a paste with rice flour (1 tsp), lemon juice (½ tsp) and fresh desi gulab petals (8–10). Apply the scrub on your face and neck while gently massaging the skin. Let it dry for five minutes. Wash off with lukewarm water.

(by Kshama Shamsukha)

- **Desi gulab and avocado hair pack:** Take half an avocado (with the rest, you can make guacamole) and mash it together with a fistful of desi gulab petals to make a thick paste. You can add olive oil (1 tsp) if you wish. Massage this on to your scalp and spread it across the strands. Wrap the head with a cotton towel dipped in hot water and leave it on for twenty minutes. Rinse off the pack and then shampoo as usual.

- **Desi gulab and sugar body polish:** Mix together coconut oil (1 tbsp), sweet almond oil (1 tbsp), small-grain white/brown sugar (7–10 tbsp) and fresh desi gulab petals (2 tbsp), or use dried petals (2 tbsp) if you want to store for longer time. Store in a glass jar. Use as an exfoliator as and when required.

(by Sangeeta Jain)

- **Gulab jal:** Take desi gulab petals (3 cups), wash and leave them on a clean cotton cloth to allow them to drain. Put the petals into a saucepan and fill the pan with distilled water till the petals are just covered. Cover the pan and heat on very low flame until most of the colour has faded from the petals. Strain, cool and store in a glass bottle.

(by Sangeeta Jain)

HIBISCUS

Known as jaba in Bengali, this vibrant flower has numerous beauty benefits. Being rich in vitamin C it boosts collagen production, thus helping in brightening and firming skin. It also nourishes and strengthens hair roots. In fact, the famous Jabakusum oil has been an essential part of Bengali households as well as a Bengali bride's wedding trousseau. According to Dr Chatterjee, hibiscus-infused oil can be excellent for hair regrowth and the paste of the flower can be used as a natural hair dye.

- **Jaba-infused coconut oil:** This recipe is my take on the flower-infused oil. In one cup of coconut oil add one cup of fresh jaba buds and store it in a transparent jar. Keep it in sunlight for 4–5 weeks, stirring the contents once a day. Then strain the oil and store it in a dark bottle. You may add a few drops of rosemary and ginger essential oils if you wish. Take a teaspoon of this oil and massage it on to the scalp, spreading it across the lengths. Keep it on for twenty minutes and then shampoo as usual.
- **Jaba and brown rice face pack:** Make a paste with cooked brown rice (2 tbsp), honey (2 tsp), geranium (4 drops) and tea tree essential oils (4 drops) and fresh jaba petals (½ cup). Apply the pack on your face and leave it on for fifteen minutes. Rinse off with lukewarm water. This face pack deep-cleans the skin and helps fight acne.

- **Jaba and coffee hair dye:** I love to colour my hair in shades of red and often highlight strands in ruby hues. In between my hair-colour sessions, once a week, I nourish my hair with this mask, which stimulates the scalp, promotes hair growth and leaves a rich auburn shade on the strands. And the hair smells divine. Overnight, steep a glass of water with a cinnamon stick. The following day boil this water with instant coffee (1 tbsp) and jaba powder (2 tbsp). Simmer it till it forms a thick paste. Cool it down to room temperature and apply this paste on your hair lengths from root to tip. Put on a shower cap and leave it for forty-five minutes. Rinse off and shampoo as usual.

MARIGOLD

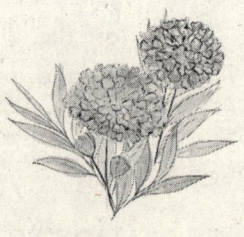

This quintessential India flower is popularly known as geinda and is known for its ability to fight acne, deep-clean skin pores and brighten complexion. It also adds shine and health to your hair.

- **Geinda and haldi brightening mask:** For glowing, clear skin, mix together grated, fresh haldi (2 tsp), marigold petals (½ cup) and fresh cream (1 tbsp). Massage this on face and neck for five minutes and leave it on for fifteen minutes. Wash off with lukewarm water.
- **Geinda-infused oil:** In a glass jar, take rosehip oil (1 cup), add geinda petals (1 cup) and fresh haldi (½ inch) and let it infuse for 3–4 weeks. Keep it in sunlight during the day and shake the jar once a day to

allow all the ingredients to mull and blend. Strain out the oil into a dark glass bottle and add orange essential oil (3–4 drops). Use this as a night oil for soft, glowing skin.

- **Geinda and neem hair rinse:** Boil beer (2 cups) with a fistful of neem leaves and fresh marigold petals (1 cup). Strain and cool it to room temperature. After shampooing your hair, use this as a final rinse for your hair. This rinse adds shine and bounce to the hair.

- **Geinda and orange body scrub:** To remove tan and exfoliate skin, especially elbows, knuckles, ankles and heels, make a scrub with coconut oil (1 cup), orange peel powder (1 tbsp), geinda petals (1 cup) and sugar (½ cup). Massage this on damp skin for ten minutes and then shower.

- **Geinda, aloe vera and sandalwood mask:** A mask with these three ingredients can treat dark spots, pimple marks and pigmentation. Grind together marigold petals (1 cup), aloe vera gel (½ cup) and sandalwood powder (1 tbsp) in a food processor. Apply it soon after you grind it. Keep it on for twenty minutes before washing it off.

(by Aparna Gupta, beauty writer)

BUTTERFLY PEA

The humble aprajita (blue peony) flower has suddenly come into the limelight and is being considered as an exotic bloom. Traditionally offered to Goddess Kali, this flower is found in abundance near temples in Calcutta. So, not so exotic for me. It is often used in Ayurvedic treatments for its cooling effect on the circulatory and nervous systems.

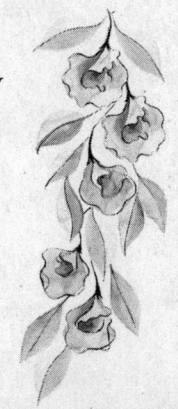

- **Aprajita and black tea hair dye:** To give your hair a deep indigo glow, make a strong cup of tea liquor with black tea leaves (2 tbsp). Strain out the tea leaves and add fresh/dry aprajita flowers (1 cup) to the liquor. Simmer it for ten minutes. Let it cool and then run it through a food processor to get a smooth paste. Apply it on your hair, starting from the roots and carefully going down to the tips. Leave it on for forty-five minutes. Rinse off and shampoo as usual.
- **Aprajita and aloe vera gel mask:** Make a paste with aloe vera gel (1 tbsp) and aprajita flowers (1 tbsp). You may add to it lavender and/or tea tree essential oil/s (2–3 drops). Apply it on your face and leave it on for forty-five minutes. You can even sleep wearing it. Wash off with splashes of water. This is excellent for soothing acne-prone skin.

LOTUS

This versatile Indian flower has several beauty benefits. Popularly known as kamal or padma, the lotus contains linoleic acid along with several other nutrients that make it an ideal ingredient for balancing the skin's sebum production, brightening complexion and hydrating skin.

- **Lotus and coconut face oil:** In a 100 ml transparent glass jar, infuse coconut oil (you can use jojoba, olive or avocado oil, or a blend of all these oils as well) with a cup of fresh lotus petals. Let it rest for 4–6 weeks. Keep it in sunlight every day and shake it up once a day. After the resting period, strain out the oil and add 2–4 drops of blue lotus essential oil. You can use it as a face massage oil.

- **Lotus, milk and honey face pack:** For an even skin tone and glow, blend together lotus petals (1 cup), milk powder (1 tbsp), milk (2 tbsp) and honey (2 tsp) in a food processor. Apply this pack on clean skin and leave it on for 15–20 minutes. Gently massage the skin while washing it off from the face.

- **Lotus and oatmeal body scrub:** Combine together equal quantities of lotus petals (you can slice them in small pieces), oatmeal and milk. Squish it all together and give your body a nice rub-down with this scrub. Rinse off with lukewarm water.

CALENDULA

Touted now as one of the most healing and nourishing oils, calendula has for ages been used for its curative properties. Sangeeta Jain, co-founder, RAS Luxury Oils, who works extensively with calendula, points out that this flower has been used in several homeopathic preparations. According to Jain, calendula oil is so gentle and conditioning that it can also be used to massage newborn babies.

- **Calendula and *manjishtha* face oil:** Mix calendula flowers (1 cup) and one pinch manjishtha powder in jojoba oil (1 cup). Keep the mix in the sun for 4–6 weeks to infuse the flowers and manjishtha. After the petals have been infused, strain out the oil into a dark glass bottle. Add manuka (20 drops) and immortelle essential oil (20 drops), shake well and use.

(*by Vasudha Rai, author of* Glow: Indian Foods, Recipes and Rituals for Beauty, Inside and Out*)*

- **Calendula face cream:** To make calendula-infused oil, take dried calendula flowers in a glass jar. Then fill it with almond oil till the petals are immersed completely. Close the lid and keep it in a warm, dark place. Shake every day for five to six weeks. Strain the oil into another fresh glass jar. Mix 150 gm of this calendula-infused oil with 50 gm sweet almond oil, 75 gm shea butter and 50 gm cocoa butter in a small bowl in a double boiler, on a low flame. As the ingredients start melting, stir well for fifteen minutes on a low flame. Transfer the contents into a glass jar; let it cool and set.

(by Sangeeta Jain)

JASMINE

This popular fragrant bloom is extensively used for its gorgeous scent as well as for its hair and skin benefits. It has cooling and moisturizing properties.

- **Mogra and milk face pack:** Boil mogra flowers (1 tbsp) in milk (½ cup) with honey (1 tsp). Let it cool down and then blend it to make a thick paste. Apply on face and neck and leave it to dry for 15–20 minutes. Wash off with splashes of cold water.
- **Mogra hair rinse:** Soak a handful of mogra flowers in hot water and allow it to cool. When cooled, apply on your hair and leave it for five minutes. Rinse off with water.

(by Sangeeta Jain)

AND SOME MORE . . .

Champa and *besan* face pack: Frangipani flower, or champak, or goloncho in Bengali, makes a perfect pack for dull, dry skin. This flower, known for its regenerative characteristics, also has anti-ageing properties, thereby delaying wrinkles and fine lines. Crush champak petals (1 cup) in water (1 cup) and add besan (½ cup) to it to make a thick paste. Apply the paste on the face and let it dry. Wash with lukewarm water after fifteen minutes.

Rajnigandha and mogra body oil: Infuse one cup of rajnigandha and mogra flowers in 100 ml of olive or jojoba oil for 4–6 weeks. While you may keep it in sunlight, the way other infusions are kept, I like to keep it out under moonlight. During the day, I store it in a cool, dry and dark place. After the resting phase, strain out the flowers and use the oil after a shower every night.

Floral bath salt and scrub: Salt crystals have a natural tendency to absorb negative energy, and the blend of water and salt is a potent energy cleanser. A bath salt soak may not brighten the skin or leave it soft, but it is a super-effective in making you feel good in your skin. If you can't get to use this daily, make it a habit to use bath salts on days/evenings you are feeling lethargic or cynical. It is the quickest and easiest way to uplift your energies. What you need: ½ cup each of sea salt and Himalayan salt, and dried and crushed desi gulab petals, mogra and lavender.

In a large bowl, combine both the salts. Stir in the rose petals, jasmine flowers and lavender. Like seasoning in a dish, you can add the dried flowers as per your taste or preference. Whether you want more of rose or jasmine or lavender is your personal choice. Desi gulab is uplifting; mogra is sensual; and lavender is relaxing. Transfer the bath salts to glass containers. Add a handful of salts to hot water for bathing, and mix oil to it. This salt soak also doubles up as a scrub. Apply this in gentle circular motion on all parts of the body, except the face. It exfoliates and nourishes at the same time. The skin feels clean, soft and smooth.

(by Aparna Gupta)

Desi gulab and mogra face mist: Boil desi gulab (1 tbsp) and mogra (1 tbsp) in two glasses of water. You may add to it a few pudina leaves for a cooling effect. Strain out the flowers and let the water cool down. Store it in a dark glass spray bottle and keep it in the fridge for future use. Whenever your skin feels tired, spritz this fragrant mist.

Lotus and desi gulab pack: To cool down inflammations and detoxify the skin, mix dried and powdered lotus petals (2 tsp) with rose water (1 tsp) to make a thick paste. Apply it on face and neck and let it dry for fifteen minutes. Wash off with splashes of water.

(by Dr Sharad Kulkarni)

PART 5

FOODS & FLAVOURS

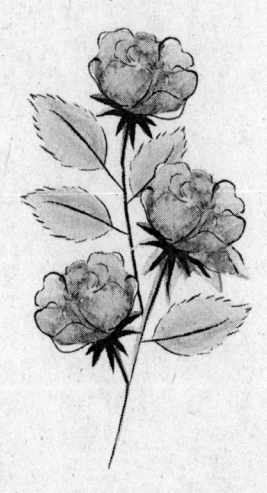

WHY EAT FLOWERS?

You would have observed pansy, borage blossoms, nasturtium or chives daintily placed on gourmet platters. I was absolutely fascinated by the dishes, or rather the plating, when I watched the first season of *MasterChef Australia*. They just made the dish look so much more appetizing. At the same time, it also made me wonder whether I should be eating these flowers. Are flowers meant for simple dressing-up of foods, or can they be eaten?

My friend and nutritionist Kavita Devgan, the author of the wonderful book *Ultimate Grandmother Hacks: 50 Kickass Traditional Habits for a Fitter You*, says that not much data is available on the nutritional value of flowers. There is confusion about which flowers are edible and which are potentially dangerous. Sometimes it is also difficult to differentiate between two varieties of blooms. They may seem similar but you can't really be sure. This lack of accessible information of edible flowers could perhaps be the reason why you wouldn't necessarily picture flowers when you think of food.

However, flowers do have nutrients in them. Dr Kaushik Majumdar, associate professor of pathology at G.B. Pant Institute of Postgraduate Medical Education and Research (GIPMER), has extensively helped me in understanding the nutritional value of flowers and patiently encouraged me in my experiments with flower essences. He explained to me that flowers get their gorgeous colours from nitrogen-rich proteins like carotenes, xanthophylls, anthocyanins and porphyrins. Speaking to him, I realized that consuming flowers could indeed be a great way of ingesting some important nutrients. In fact, the reason you should include flowers in your diet is the same reason why you would have colourful veggies in your diet.

In my experiments cooking with flowers I have realized that the best use of highly pigmented flowers is to use them as food colouring. I like to use fresh flowers for creating the colour.

To begin with, I thoroughly wash the flowers with water and alcohol. After straining out the excess water, I take out the petals and then boil them in drinking water for about ten minutes and then let it rest for another 10–15 minutes. Post that, I strain out the water and make a paste with the residue petals. I add this paste back to the water. This colour-concentrated water can be used in the place of synthetic food colouring to create different rice preparations, syrups, sugar or salt crystals, batters, ice creams, sauces, preserves and curries.

FLOWERS IN OUR KITCHEN

While eating flowers may seem somewhat exotic, in reality we have been eating quite a few flowers in our meals. The humble cauliflower and broccoli, and the pineapple (a combination of several flowerets), and some spices like clove/laung, saffron/kesar, star anise and mace/*javitri* are all flowers used extensively in flavouring dishes.

COOKING WITH FLOWERS

I grew up in a Bengali household where several dishes have the flower as its hero. Banana flower, or *mocha* as it is called in Bengali, is used to cook a delicacy with prawns. Incidentally, mocha can't be eaten on Tuesdays and Saturdays. My maternal grandmother used to make fritters with pumpkin flowers, and my cook makes similar fritters with ridge gourd flowers. Drumstick flowers are also cooked in Bengali and Sindhi cuisine. Here are some popular recipes that are cooked in the kitchens of my friends and family.

SWANJHRO JA GUL BY VARUN RANA

Varun is a dear friend. He is a fashion journalist and a great cook. His gastronomic initiative #RanaKaKhana has quickly become the talk of the town. My conversations with Varun almost always focus on food and emotions; hence, recipes from him had to be a part of this book.

In the winter, the drumstick trees burst into snow-white and light-yellow blossoms, which, Varun says, 'are a favourite of the Sindhi community'. While growing up, a Sindhi friend of his mother's used to cook these delicate flowers into a curry that looked and tasted like a hearty keema, but was actually what we would today call 'vegan'. 'There's no milk or animal fat used in this, and of course, no meat. Just these wonderful flowers and our amazing Indian spices and condiments,' Varun explains.

Varun's advice: Be prepared, this is not an easy recipe. The more love you put into this recipe, the better it will taste.

Below are the basic steps for preparing the flowers for cooking; this is for about 1 kg of flowers, which will reduce in volume after we boil them:

1. Buying the flowers: In the markets, the bunches of drumstick flowers you get will mostly be buds . . . but try to get your hands on a bunch that has more bloomed flowers.

2. Cleaning the flowers: Drumstick flowers have thin stems that are extremely bitter, so those have to be removed individually from each flower, with lots of care and attention.

3. Preparing the flowers: The flowers and buds themselves are bitter, and need to be boiled and drained at least three times before you can begin the real cooking. So in a large, deep pan, bring water (5 litres) to a boil and add salt (1 tbsp). Add in the cleaned flowers and boil for five minutes or so. Drain the flowers in a big sieve for five minutes, till the excess water runs off. Repeat this process two more times, making it a total of three boil-and-drain cycles.

4. Squeezing the flowers: Once the flowers have drained and cooled after the third (and last) boiling, squeeze the water out of them thoroughly. Now the flowers are ready for cooking. These can be stored in the fridge for about a week or so.

Ingredients:

2 onions finely chopped
1 inch of ginger grated or smashed into a paste
5–6 cloves of garlic grated or smashed into a paste

2 green chillies slit lengthwise
2 cups tomato puree or grated tomatoes
½ cup dahi
¼ tbsp haldi powder
¼ tbsp garam masala
½ tbsp *lal mirch* powder
½ tbsp *dhania* powder
Salt to taste (you have boiled the flowers in salted water already, so add salt in the end after tasting, and if required)
3–4 tbsp oil for cooking (I use mustard oil, but you can use normal cooking oil as well. If using mustard oil, heat the oil in the cooking pan till it begins to smoke, and then turn off the flame. Let it cool for 2–3 minutes and then light the flame again to begin cooking)

Method:

1) Heat the oil on high flame, and add in the finely chopped onions and sauté till they are translucent and well-sweated.
2) Add in the ginger and garlic paste and sauté till they don't smell raw any more.
3) Add in the green chillies and sauté well; turn the flame to low.
4) Add in powdered spices and give a quick stir; you don't want to burn them in the hot oil.
5) Immediately add in the prepared flowers and mix well. Cook on medium flame till the water evaporates completely and the flowers become fluffy.

6) Add in the dahi and tomato puree, and cook on low flame (stirring frequently) till the tomatoes don't smell raw any more, and leave the oil at the edges of the pan.

7) You can also add peas to this, if you like.

8) Taste and add salt as per your taste.

9) Garnish with chopped coriander stems (not leaves; the stems have the most flavour) and serve hot with *bajre ki* roti or simple roti, whichever you prefer.

SHOJNEPHOOL'ER POSTO BY RUBY BISWAS

My mother, Ruby Biswas, is one of the most talented women that I have ever come across. She is a renowned make-up artist and the first woman in our family to make a career of her own. Of the many things she excels in, cooking is surely one of her best skills. The book would remain incomplete without contributions from her.

Much before drumstick flowers acquired the cult status of a super-food, *shojnephool* (or what Varun calls in Sindhi, *swanjhro ja gul*) was a humble staple in our kitchen. My mother uses drumsticks and its flowers extensively. While the drumsticks or *shojne danta* were used to make *shukto* (a kind of bitter veg stew) and *chanchra* (a type of mixed vegetables cooked with fish head), shojne flowers (phool) were used to make *chorchori* (which is the next recipe) or *posto*. Now, of course, she also steeps the flowers in warm water and drinks it first thing in the morning to keep her blood sugar in control.

Before moving on with the recipe, let me tell you a little about posto. What is posto? It is basically poppy seeds or khuskhus. It is a Bengali delicacy. A creamy paste made of ground posto and water is used in various combinations to make several dishes. It is cooked with potatoes to make the famous *aloo posto*, with egg to make *deem posto*, with ridge gourd to make *jheenge posto* and so on. Shojnephool'er posto is one of these many variations of posto.

Like Varun, my mother also avoids the shojne buds and picks out the bloomed flowers as the buds can be bitter. She does not boil the flowers but washes them in a sieve under running water.

The posto paste can be made in two ways. One is the traditional method of soaking the posto in water, washing it thoroughly and then straining out the excess water. These soaked grains are then used to make a butter-like, creamy paste with a traditional *silbatta/sheelnora*. You can try a granite mortar and pestle for the same, but I prefer the paste that my cook makes with sheelnora. My mother-in-law, however, employs a simpler technique. She washes and cleans the posto, as my mother does, but grinds it in a blender. This technique is definitely far easier and works better when making a larger quantity of paste. So she makes the paste and keeps it refrigerated up to seven days.

Ingredients:

2 tbsp posto paste
250 gm fresh shojne flowers
1 tbsp mustard oil
1 big potato diced
1 medium-sized onion diced
2 green chillies finely chopped
¼ tsp haldi powder
Pinch of lal mirch powder
Salt to taste

Method:

1) Marinade potato with haldi, salt and lal mirch.
2) In a kadai heat half of the mustard oil on high flame till it smokes. Then reduce the flame to low.
3) Sauté the potato in this oil and keep it aside.
4) Add the remaining oil in the kadai and fry the diced onion till it turns translucent.
5) Put in shojnephool, potato and green chillies, and stir a little. Add posto, salt and water.
6) Close with a lid and let it cook till the water dries out, and till potatoes and flowers are soft and the posto has a creamy texture.
7) Serve with warm rice and *gondhoraj* lime.

SHOJNE PHOOL'ER CHORCHORI BY BUTA BERA

My cook and housekeeper Buta is one of the most caring souls around me. She cooks with a lot of love and is forever indulging and pampering me with the amazing food that she cooks. When Buta got to know that I am writing a book, she was super-excited and did whatever she could to help me with the same—cups of tea and coffee, a neck and shoulder massage, applying hair packs, helping out with trying out various recipes, and running my home in such a way that I didn't have to look into day-to-day things.

Though thrilled, she shared this recipe with a lot of apprehension about whether it would be liked by the readers.

So before we move on to the dish, allow me to explain what a chorchori is. It is a Bengali version of mixed vegetable and is a dry preparation. In Bengali cuisine there are different variations of mixed veggies; the difference primarily lies in the spices that are used in it. In chorchori, a very indigenous five-spice mix called '*paanchphoron*', that includes jeera, methi, saunf, *kala* jeera and *radhuni* (it is similar to celery seeds; sometimes it is replaced with mustard seeds), is used.

Buta does not boil the shojne flowers. She cleans and washes them well, strains out the excess water and mixes the blooms with haldi, lal mirch and salt and keeps it aside before starting to cook.

Ingredients:

500 gm fresh shojnephool
1 big potato diced
2 big onions finely chopped
1 tsp paanchphoron
1 lal mirch
¼ tsp lal mirch powder
2 tsp mustard paste
¼ tsp haldi powder
Salt to taste
2 tbsp mustard oil
5 *bori* (optional)
10 shrimps (optional; if you decide to add the shrimps, you can marinate them with a pinch of salt and haldi powder)

Method:

1) Heat oil on high flame and when it starts to smoke, reduce the flame and add paanchphoron. Stir it for a minute.

2) Put in the diced onions, followed by the potato.
3) Cover and cook for about 15–20 minutes, stirring it from time to time till the potato cubes soften.
4) Add the marinated flowers and keep stirring for ten minutes. Then take it off the flame.
5) Separately fry bori and/or shrimps and sprinkle it over the chorchori.
6) Eat with rice, dal, fresh green chilli and a sprinkle of lemon juice.

KUMRO PHOOL'ER PAKORA BY NAMITA GHOSH

Namita Ghosh was my late grandmother and best friend. She was very petite and quiet but was quite a silent dynamite. She never complained, never shouted, but held a storm within and it would roll out when she cooked. I feel she just didn't 'love' food; rather, she had a torrid affair with it. Her relationship with different foods was pronounced. For instance, she hated dhania with a vengeance but loved curry leaves passionately.

Watching her cook made me happy and I acquired the sharp tastes she had. One of her favourite dishes was pumpkin flower fritters or *kumro phool'er* pakora. I remember the first time I saw these bright yellow flowers I fell in love with them. They looked so beautiful. With a deep fascination I watched my grandmother carefully wash them, cut out the petals and then leave them aside to drain out the extra water, before frying them.

I try to make these pakoras when I miss her. It's difficult to get these blooms in the market and so I have planted two pumpkin creepers to supply me with the flowers.

Ingredients:

10–12 pumpkin flowers
2 tbsp besan
1 tsp rice flour
1 green chilli finely chopped
½ tsp kala jeera
¼ tsp haldi powder
Pinch of lal mirch powder
3 tbsp mustard oil
Salt as per taste
Water as needed

Method:

1) Mix together besan, rice flour, green chilli, lal mirch powder, kala jeera, haldi and salt with water to create a batter that's neither too thick nor too thin/runny—just thick enough to coat the petals with a thin layer.

2) Heat the oil in a deep kadai.

3) Dip each petal at a time in the batter; shake off the excess batter and then put it into the oil for frying. Repeat with all the petals.

4) Fry them golden and then take them off the kadai and place them over paper towels to absorb the excess oil.

5) Serve with spicy chutney as a snack or as a side dish with khichdi. You can also have it with plain rice and dal.

KUMRO PHOOL'ER TAK BY BUTA BERA

'*Tak*' in Bengali means 'sour'. And in Bengali cuisine it means a sour curry. There are numerous variations of this curry. One can make it with tamarind and hilsa, bhindi and lemon, aloo, *baigan* and raw mango, and many more. Buta loves to make these sour curries on days she's very tired. Among my many favourites is this one she makes with pumpkin flowers.

Ingredients:

12 pumpkin flowers
2 lal mirch
1 tsp paanchphoron
½ tsp sugar
2 tsp white mustard seed or paste
2 tsp aamchoor
2 tsp mustard oil
A pinch of salt

Preparation: Clean pumpkin flowers, remove the petals and wash them well; mix with haldi and lal mirch powder.

Method:

1) In hot oil put paanchphoron and lal mirch.
2) Add the petals and stir.
3) Add 1 cup water and simmer.
4) Add salt, mustard paste and sugar.
5) Add aamchoor and simmer.
6) Serve it with plain rice and a green chilli.

KACHNAAR KI KALI KA ACHAAR BY VARUN RANA

This is another recipe by Varun. It is quite tedious but extremely delicious. Here's what he has to say about the achaar/pickle. I am quoting him below because of the poetic way he has described the flowers and the method of cooking.

'One of the most beautiful sights of autumn is the blooming of bauhinias across north India. You may know it as mountain ebony, and in Hindi we call them by the charming name of *kachnaar*. The trees shed all their leaves, and the flowers take over, setting the tree ablaze with their lovely, distinct lavender hue.

'Right before the buds burst into bloom, I like to pick them and pickle them. They have a distinct sour flavour, and a slight tannin that makes you want to go back for more. I learnt this from my Himachali aunt, whose house in Baijnath has a garden full of these beautiful trees.'

Ingredients:

1 kg kachnaar buds
50 gm turmeric powder
40 gm red chilli powder
50 gm salt
75 gm powdered mustard seeds
1 litre mustard oil (heat this in a pan till it begins smoking, and then turn off the flame and let it cool down)

Preparing the kachnaar buds:

These can be bitter and dirty, so spend some time preparing them to be pickled. Here's how:

1) In a large pan, pour about 1.5 litres of water at room temperature, add 2–3 tbsp of salt, and soak the buds in the solution for about three hours.
2) Drain the salt water and wash the buds in fresh, flowing water.
3) In a large pan, bring 2 litres of water to a roaring boil, and add in the buds. Take them out in about thirty seconds maximum.
4) Spread them on a clean sheet and dry them in the sun for about 5–6 hours.

Method:

1) In a big kadai, heat the burnt-and-cooled mustard oil.
2) Add in the salt, turmeric and red chilli powder. Immediately turn off the flame. Mix well so that no lumps may form.
3) Add the kachnaar buds and mix well, and set aside to cool down.
4) Once cooled, add in the mustard seed/rai powder, and mix well.
5) Transfer this into big, airtight glass jars, and sun them for a week to ten days; the gentle heat of the sun helps the spices to permeate the buds, after which the pickle will be ready to eat.

MOCHA CHINGRI'R TORKARI BY RUBY BISWAS

Mocha is banana flower. *Chingri* refers to the entire genre of shrimps, prawns and lobsters. In this very popular dish, shrimps are used. Whenever I visit Kolkata, mocha chingri has to be a part of at least one of my meals. My mother makes several preparations with mocha; however, I like this one the best. Like kachnaar and shojnephool, mocha takes time and patience to prepare for cooking.

Preparing the mocha: Cleaning the mocha flowers is the most difficult part of this recipe.

1) Apply some mustard oil on your hands before starting to separate the flowers, as the banana flowers can stain your hands.

2) Remove each red petal or bract and collect the florets or tiny bananas. Continue to do this until you reach the inner part where there are no more bracts to be removed and there's a yellowish bulb-like centre.

3) Each floweret will have one stamen with a small head and a transparent plastic-like covering. Remove them and discard.

4) Bunch all the florets together and chop into fine pieces. Put them in a bowl filled with two cups of water.

5) Add to this water a pinch of salt and turmeric powder; pressure-cook the flowers for one whistle.

6) Drain out the water and the flowers are ready to be cooked.

Ingredients:

2 cups boiled banana flowers mixed with turmeric powder and salt
1 big potato diced and mixed with turmeric powder and salt

1 cup shrimps peeled, cleaned, deveined and mixed with turmeric powder and salt
1½ tbsp mustard oil
2 tsp ghee
2 tsp onion paste
1 tsp ginger paste
1 tsp jeera powder
1 tomato diced
2 green chillies chopped
1 small cinnamon stick
4 cloves
3 cardamoms
1 *tejpatta*
1 lal mirch
1 tsp garam masala powder
1 tsp sugar
¼ tsp lal mirch powder
2 tsp turmeric powder
1 cup grated coconut
Salt as per taste

Method:

1) Warm oil and ghee together in a kadai till the ghee lets off its fragrance.
2) Sauté shrimps and keep them aside.
3) Sauté potato and keep it aside.
4) Put in tejpatta, lal mirch, cinnamon, clove, cardamom and let it splutter.
5) Add chopped onion and fry till translucent.

6) Stir in ginger paste, tomato, haldi powder, jeera powder and lal mirch powder. Keep stirring till oil starts separating.

7) Add boiled mocha, potato and shrimps.

8) Add sugar; cover and cook till it is soft and dry.

9) Garnish with grated coconut and serve with boiled rice.

PHOOLKOPI'R MALAI CURRY BY ARPITA CHATTERJEE

Arpita Chatterjee is my sister. She is a compassionate and patient homemaker, a respected and well-loved teacher, and an excellent cook. Bengali and Anglo-Indian cuisines and bakery are her forte.

So what is 'phoolkopi'? It is cauliflower; and 'malai curry' literally means cream curry. In Bengali fare, prawn malai curry is a delicacy and the phoolkopi'r malai curry is generally seen as its insipid veg cousin. However, my sister's phoolkopi'r malai curry is a different story.

At a recent dinner at her place she had prepared both the veg and non-veg versions of the curry, and I had laughed and said, 'Who will eat phoolkopi when there's chingri on the table?' I had to eat my words and both versions of the malai curry, and admit that, despite the chingri malai curry being excellent, she had beaten it with her phoolkopi number. Needless to say the phoolkopi got consumed at the dinner and the chingri was left over and served as our lunch the next day.

Ingredients:

1 cauliflower
1 tbsp green peas
250 ml coconut milk
1 tbsp onion paste
1 tsp ginger paste
2 cinnamon sticks
5–6 cloves
2 cardamoms smashed
1 tejpatta
2 lal mirch
1 pinch lal mirch powder
1 pinch turmeric powder
½ tsp sugar

Method:

1) Chop the cauliflower into small pieces.
2) Lightly fry the cauliflower and peas till almost cooked. Keep aside.
3) Heat oil in a kadai.
4) Add the sugar. As soon as it caramelizes, add red chillies, cinnamon, cardamom and cloves.
5) The aroma of the spices will come forth. Immediately, add onion paste and ginger paste.
6) Fry well until oil leaves the sides and the paste is brown in colour.
7) Add the red chilli powder, diluted in a little bit of water, and the turmeric.

8) When the oil starts separating, add the coconut milk.
9) Bring the gravy to a boil.
10) Add the fried cauliflower and peas, and cook in the gravy for about fifteen minutes.
11) Check to see if it is soft and cooked.
12) Can be served with plain rice but tastes best when had with *luchi* (Bengali version of puri made with refined flour) or *koraishuti'r kochuri* (peas kachori).

FLOWERS IN GOURMET FOOD

While writing this book I had reached out to friends, family and professional chefs for recipes. Friends and relatives graciously contributed, and I have also been indulged by professional chefs who have very kindly shared some of their recipes and their culinary skills with me.

FLOWER FAIRY'S KITCHEN

Chef Radhika Khandelwal dishes out some of the prettiest meals from her restaurant, Fig & Maple. If you have not seen the Instagram account @figandmaple of this place, do it now. It is a delight to just see the plates. It looks as if a fairy has visited the kitchen.

Radhika discovered her passion for cooking while pursuing a course in hairdressing in Melbourne, and I guess her love for fresh produce and style of plating seem influenced by her time there.

She tells me that, in India, roses and *kewda* flowers in particular have been used for their flavouring and colouring properties since the Mughal era. There was no feast without the flavouring of the above mentioned.

Radhika extensively uses edible flowers such as pansies, pumpkin flowers, zucchini flowers, carnations, lilacs, hibiscuses, banana blossoms, sunflowers, nasturtiums, marigolds, basil flowers, carrot flowers, frangipanis, butterfly peas, dianthuses and even the inside bud of bougainvilleas seasonally in her daily cooking at her restaurant. 'The flavours of a particular dish can be heightened extensively by using the correct flower with the correct dish, which also adds a visual treat to the eyes,' she says.

To bring out the best of each flower's flavours and properties, Radhika suggests one segregate flowers into different sections. For instance, she uses hibiscus, basil, onion flower, marigold and rose to create syrups, jams, infusions and pastes. Whereas pansies, carrot flowers and dianthuses are used for garnishing salads, soups, mains and some desserts. She uses some flowers like butterfly peas for their medicinal properties and natural colouring in certain dishes and drinks on her menu.

Nasturtiums and zucchini flowers are very versatile and are used as dishes themselves—such as fritters and salads. Nasturtiums, being extremely peppery in flavour, add a lot of zing to a dish. Those who want to experiment a little with their food can perhaps begin with these flower fritters.

Radhika has shared with me two of her very stylish and delicate dishes. I believe that what you cook reflects the kind of person you are. Radhika's gentle personality shines through the food she brings to the table. What I loved about her contribution was that she was sensitive to the fact that I am a Bengali and came up with recipes especially for this book, where Bengali culinary elements like banana flowers, *gondhorajlebu*, *nolengur*, prawns and aprajita blossoms were presented with a modern twist.

BANANA BLOSSOM SALAD

Ingredients for salad:

2 banana flowers
1 gondhorajlebu
6 tiger prawns peeled, cleaned and cooked with tails intact
2 spring onions thinly sliced
1 bunch coriander
1 red onion thinly sliced
1 red pepper thinly sliced
1 yellow pepper thinly sliced

Ingredients for dressing:

2 tbsp tamarind
1 tbsp lime juice
1 tbsp nolengur extract
2 tbsp coconut cream
1 tbsp fish sauce

Method:

1) Remove purple outer coverings from the banana flower, and discard the paper-like cover and sticky structure; you should be left with only the very tender, off-white florets. All other parts of the banana flower are to be discarded.

2) Place the florets in a bowl with a solution of 2 litres water, lemon juice and 1 tbsp salt to prevent browning. Halve the banana blossom cores, slice diagonally and add to the acidulated water. You can also place them in buttermilk for the same effect.

3) To make the dressing, mix all ingredients together. Taste to balance.

4) For the salad, toss all ingredients, including the cleaned banana florets, together in a bowl. Add dressing to taste. Mix well. Serve.

BUTTERFLY PEA SPRITZER

Ingredients for syrup:

½ cup of butterfly pea flowers (aprajita)
½ cup water
½ cup sugar

Make a simple syrup with water and sugar and add the aprajita flowers in the syrup. Your syrup is ready to be used in drinks and food.

Ingredients for spritzer:

60 ml vodka
15 ml aprajita syrup
10 ml lemon juice
Ice as required
60 ml sparkling wine
Soda to top

Method:

1) In a spritzer glass add the vodka, butterfly pea syrup, lemon juice and ice.
2) Top the glass with sparkling wine and soda, and the spritzer is ready to serve.

FROM THE FLOWER GARDEN TO THE GOURMET TABLE

One of the best things about Pullman Aerocity, Delhi, is their restaurant, Pluck, where their seasonal menu includes the fresh produce from their in-house farm. The hotel's Director of Culinary, Chef Ajay Anand, has rustled up a flavourful and exclusive dish for this book.

While working on this particular recipe, his primary focus was to use a local Indian flower which is a significant part of our culture. 'So I picked the gorgeous marigold flower,' he says. 'Wherever you go, you will find this beautiful flower with its lovely appearance and fragrance,' Chef Anand explains. Making the vibrant bloom the hero of the dish, he uses it in cooking as well as for plating the same.

MARIGOLD PESTO WITH BASIL CRUMBLE AND TOMATO TEA

Ingredients for marigold pesto:

200 gm freshly plucked marigold flowers
2 gm green chilli

2 gm ginger
10 gm garlic
20 gm Parmesan cheese
25 gm cashew nut
Salt to taste
50 ml olive oil

Ingredients for basil crumble:

100 gm fresh basil
50 gm unsalted butter
50 gm multigrain flour
10 ml milk
20 ml chlorophyll oil
Salt a pinch
2 gm black peppercorn crushed

Ingredients for tomato tea:

500 gm fresh plum tomatoes
10 gm garlic
10 gm coriander roots
Salt to taste
10 ml white balsamic vinegar
3 gm castor sugar

Method for marigold pesto:

1) Cut marigold flower buds and remove the stem part; reserve only petals.

2) Wash petals thoroughly and blanch it for two seconds; this is the most important part as we don't want to lose any of its flavour. We only want to make it soft.

3) Plunge the petals in the ice water, drain it well and squeeze to get rid of excess moisture.

4) In a blender put all the ingredients, except oil and cheese. Blend it to a smooth texture; avoid over-blending, which might discolour the puree.

5) Fold in the olive oil and Parmesan cheese. Strain the mixture through a fine strainer.

Method for basil crumble:

1) Pluck basil leaves and discard the stems. Wash thoroughly and pat dry the same.

2) Blanch the leaves and blend to a thick paste.

3) In a bowl, mix multigrain flour and cold butter; mix slowly with your fingertips to a breadcrumb texture.

4) Add milk, salt and basil paste to the above mix to make dough; avoid over-kneading.

5) Roll the dough and bake it at 60 degrees Celsius for around 100 minutes.

6) Crumble the above sheet to a powder.

Method for tomato tea:

1) Wash tomatoes; cut them into quarters. In a centrifugal juicer take out tomato juice along with garlic and coriander roots.

2) Boil the juice on high flame and let it simmer. Discard the scum and keep only clear water at the bottom.

3) Season the same with white balsamic vinegar, salt and castor sugar.

Final Plate-up:

In a bowl make a dollop of marigold pesto, sprinkle basil crumble and garnish the same with marigold flower petals. Serve tomato tea on the side.

OLD WORLD GOURMET

Indian Habitat Centre (IHC), New Delhi, has a classic charm about everything it contains. I love the food at its restaurants as they have an old-world appeal. In fact, I particularly like the fare at the Oriental Octopus—specifically, their rose petal ice cream. At my request, Rajiv Malhotra, Corporate Chef, Habitat World, IHC, has shared the recipe of this dessert, along with that of Delhi 'O' Delhi's *dahi gulkand kebab*.

DAHI GULKAND KEBAB

Ingredients:

1 kg dahi
5 gm cardamom powder
10 gm white pepper powder
10 gm green chillies chopped
10 gm ginger chopped

100 gm cornflour
Salt to taste
Oil for frying

Ingredients for gulkand:

250 gm rose petals
250 gm granulated sugar

Making gulkand: Wash the rose petals, and drain and wipe them with a clean cloth. Chop roughly and keep aside; then take a glass jar and put one layer of petals and top with equal amount of sugar. Repeat the process till all the ingredients are used. Cover the jar with a lid and place under sunlight for 7–10 days.

Stir the mixture with a spoon once a day to ensure that both the items are mixed evenly. Store in refrigerator when done.

Method:

1) In a muslin cloth, pour the yogurt and hang overnight to remove excess whey.
2) In a clean glass bowl, take the overnight hung curd, add half of the chopped green chillies, ginger, cardamom powder, salt and cornflour. Mix well and divide into individual kebab-like portions and keep aside.
3) For making the stuffing, take some prepared gulkand and place over a sieve to drain excess moisture.
4) Pour the drained gulkand in a separate bowl and mix remaining chopped ginger and green chillies and mix well.

5) Now take the individual portions of the yogurt mixture, make a depression in the centre and place the gulkand stuffing; cover and make flat patties. Repeat till all the patties are made. Keep in refrigerator for twenty minutes.

6) Heat oil in a pan and deep-fry the patties till crisp and golden in colour.

7) Remove and serve hot with mint chutney.

ROSE PETAL ICE CREAM

Ingredients for rose syrup:

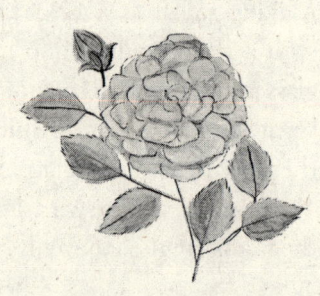

500 gm unsalted butter
250 gm bakery cream
15 gm dried rose petals
400 ml Rooh Afza syrup

Mix all together to create the rose syrup.

Ingredients for the ice cream:

4 litres vanilla ice cream
400 gm milk powder
150 gm rose syrup
10 gm dried rose petals

Method:

1) Combine all the above-mentioned ingredients together, including the rose syrup.

2) Mix until the mixture becomes smooth.
3) Pour the mixture into jars for freezing.
4) Freeze it for about 4–5 hours, until you get the correct consistency.
5) Serve in ice cream bowls.

FROM THE HIMALAYAS

Blue cheese—exotic; marigold—commonplace; but what will their union be like? Chef Diwaker, Executive Chef, Ananda in the Himalayas, offers a unique suggestion.

MARIGOLD AND BLUE CHEESE DIP

Ingredients:

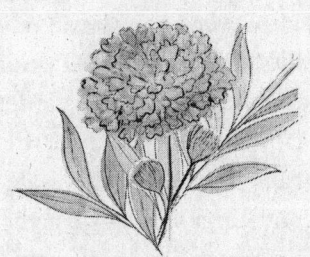

1 cup marigold leaves
1 tbsp blue cheese
1 tsp black salt
1½ tbsp brown sugar
2 tbsp soy milk
6 tbsp olive oil

Method:

1) Blend together the milk and oil.
2) Blanch geinda (marigold) petals and puree with sugar, salt and cheese.
3) Add soy milk and oil emulsion to this puree.
4) Mix well and chill.
5) Serve as a dip with bread/breadsticks.

GETTING CREATIVE WITH BLOOMS

Flowers symbolize creativity, and when you spend enough time with them, you are able to manifest your own creativity, compassion and imagination. While I have always been mesmerized by flowers, my appreciation for blooms and their many benefits has blossomed with each passing day. My culinary skills have greatly improved and the excitement with trying something new, and innovating and renovating old recipes have made my kitchen a play zone.

Along with me, some very kind friends have fired their imagination and skills to share some gorgeous new dishes and traditional recipes with a modern twist.

If you are an enthusiastic home cook, open to experiments and innovations, begin with flowers that are easily available. However, be careful about where you are procuring the blooms from. Best option is to grow them in your balcony, terrace or kitchen garden. If that's not possible, get them from the local flower vendor. Most cities have their typical early-morning wholesale flower markets. Make a trip to it once in a while—just the visit itself can be a fun trip. Avoid flowers from boutiques as they may contain preservatives. Also remember to wash flowers thoroughly before cooking them.

DESI GULAB

A natural flavouring agent high in antioxidants, a stress buster and mood enhancer, rose is best used in making syrups, jams, water infusions and rice (pulao/biryani), and in desi desserts such as kheer, *seviyaan* and gulkand. When I use rose, I always use the desi gulab or the Indian wild rose for its rich, spicy-sweet aroma. With desi gulab, I have made syrups, infusions and colouring and flavouring agents in different dishes.

ROSE AND STRAWBERRY SYRUP

Ingredients:

250 gm desi gulab petals washed, cleaned and pressed dry with a kitchen towel
10–12 strawberries diced into small pieces
2 cups sugar
3 cups water

Method:

1) Heat water and sugar in a pan and allow the sugar to dissolve completely.
2) Add the flowers and strawberries to it and let it all simmer till it reaches a consistency that you desire.
3) You may blend it to get a smooth texture.
4) Let it cool and then store in glass jars in a refrigerator.

This syrup can be used to make beverages like rose sherbet by just dissolving it with water and ice, or a milkshake, or a spritzer like the one suggested by Radhika Khandelwal. I have thickened it a little by adding cornflour to it to make a preserve.

PORK SAUSAGE IN WINE AND ROSE

This is one of my favourite winter delicacies; I love to cook it for my Christmas Eve party.

Ingredients:

1 kg fresh pork sausage
1 bottle of red wine
8–10 cloves
5–6 star anise
10–12 black peppercorns coarsely crushed
1 tsp sugar
250 gm desi gulab petals washed, cleaned and pressed dry with a kitchen towel
½ tsp cornflour mixed in 1 tbsp of warm water
Salt to taste

Method:

Put all the ingredients into a kadai and simmer it till the wine reduces to a thick, sticky gravy. You can have it as a starter or with breads or mashes.

GULAB GULAUTI KEBAB

This is an innovation I made after being inspired by the Delhi 'O' Delhi's dahi gulkand kebab. The *gulauti* kebab can be replaced by any shammi kebab, or you can order the kebab from your local eatery, if you wish to make it quick and easy.

I simply call for the buttery gulauti kebab from the famous Rajender Dhaba near my house. I mash it all up and create smaller kebab portions. I then make a small depression in the portions and stuff it with rose preserve mixed with chopped green chilli and pudina leaves. This is then cooked on a tawa with just a drop of oil.

However, if you want to make from scratch, here's a recipe of shammi kebab that I learnt from my mother-in-law, Chandra Bose, and then tweaked with my love for desi gulab.

Ingredients to flavour the meat:

½ kg mutton keema
125 gm channa dal
2 onions diced in cubes
10 garlic cloves
2 inches of ginger
1 big cardamom
6–8 black peppercorns
1 inch cinnamon stick
2 tejpatta
1 javitri
1 nutmeg
½ tsp khuskhus (poppy seeds)
50 gm desi gulab petals washed, cleaned and pressed dry with a kitchen towel
Salt to taste

Ingredients for stuffing:

1 tsp lemon juice
10–12 coriander leaves chopped
6–8 mint leaves chopped
2 green chillies chopped
½ tsp garam masala powder
1 onion finely chopped
2 tsp dried desi gulab petals crushed
3–4 strands of saffron

Method:

1) Pressure-cook the keema with all its flavouring spices till tender. Don't put much water; in fact, you can skip water as the keema and gulab will give off water.
2) If there's any water left, keep cooking it till the water evaporates.
3) Blend the mixture into a coarse paste.
4) Make small roundels of the mixture.
5) Mix all the ingredients of the stuffing and keep it aside.
6) Take each roundel at a time, make a depression in the middle, put in a little of the stuffing, and roll it up to make a round. Press it flat to form small kebabs.
7) Heat a non-stick tawa and put ½ tsp of oil on it.
8) When the oil is hot, put the kebabs on the tawa. Fry them till they are golden brown.
9) Serve either with green chutney or with Malabari paratha or *romali* roti.

CHICKEN GHEE ROAST WITH DESI GULAB

I learnt this ghee roast recipe from my cousin Snigdha Hazra. I tweaked it to create my own gulab ghee roast.

Ingredients:

1 kg chicken
250 gm desi gulab petals washed, cleaned and pressed dry with a kitchen towel
2 Kashmiri lal mirch split in two
3 tsp jeera
3 tsp dhania seeds
4 tsp Kashmiri lal mirch powder
1 inch tamarind soaked in half cup of water
½ tsp methi seeds
7–8 curry leaves
1 cup curd
1 tsp garlic paste
1 tsp ginger paste
¼ tsp haldi powder
Salt to taste
3 tbsp ghee
2 inch chunk of date jaggery or gur

Method:

1) Marinade chicken with dahi, turmeric powder, ginger paste, garlic paste and salt.
2) Roast jeera, methi, whole lal mirch, dhania, curry leaves and 100 gm of rose petals on a tawa.

3) Grind them all together.

4) Strain out the tamarind water and mix it with the ground masala to create a paste.

5) Heat ghee in a kadai and, when it warms up, add the piece of gur.

6) When the gur melts and starts bubbling, add 100 gm of rose petals and lal mirch powder.

7) When the rose gives off its aroma, stir in the masala paste. Simmer it for a minute and then add in the chicken.

8) For the first five minutes, keep stirring and mixing it all. Then cover and cook, stirring from time to time, till the chicken is cooked through and the ghee starts to separate.

9) Serve it with hot rotis or rice with a wedge of lime, onions and green chilli.

ROSE AND STRAWBERRY ICE CREAM

This recipe is inspired from the rose petal ice cream from Oriental Octopus. It is my easy take on this lovely dessert.

Ingredients:

4 tbsp rose and strawberry preserve (recipe mentioned before)
5–6 strawberries cubed
½ tin Milkmaid
100 ml coconut milk
100 ml cream
10–12 desi gulab petals washed and cleaned for decoration

Method:

1) Blend together syrup, Milkmaid, coconut milk and cream.
2) Transfer it to a bowl for setting.
3) Add in cubed strawberries.
4) Freeze it for an hour.
5) Take it out and place the fresh rose petals over it.
6) Freeze it again for another hour and your ice cream is ready to be served.

GULAB-INFUSED WHISKEY

Ingredients:

200 ml whiskey
50 gm desi gulab petals washed, cleaned and pressed dry with a kitchen towel
10 black peppercorns

Method:

1) Mix it all together and store in an airtight jar or bottle in a cool, dry place for 2–3 days.
2) Shake the jar/bottle once a day to stir up the contents within.
3) After the resting phase, strain out the liquor and discard the petals and cinnamon stick.
4) Your whiskey infusion is now ready to be served.

You can make a similar infusion with cold brew coffee instead of whiskey and you may then add Irish whiskey to it to create a cocktail.

ATTA HALWA WITH GULAB BY SHRUTI ANAND

Kada prasad or atta halwa that is offered during pujas or as a prasad in gurudwaras is a delightful dessert that has been perfected by most Punjabi homes. Shruti adds to it some desi gulab petals to make it more fragrant.

Ingredients:

2 cups water
1 cup sugar
2 tbsp fresh desi gulab petals
1 cup coarsely grounded atta
1 cup desi ghee

Method:

1) Warm water in a saucepan and add sugar and some desi gulab petals (save some for garnishing) and bring it to a boil. Keep stirring till the sugar dissolves.
2) Remove the mix from the stove and keep it aside. Strain out the petals.
3) In a kadai, warm desi ghee and atta. Let the atta bubble in ghee.
4) Stir it continuously, keeping the flame on medium. Keep cooking till it is rich brown in colour with a grainy/sandy texture.

5) Add the sugar and gulab syrup to it.
6) Continue stirring till atta absorbs the entire syrup.
7) Cook for 5–7 minutes more till the halwa gets a little thicker and the ghee starts separating.
8) Garnish with fresh desi gulab petals and serve.

LAVENDER

Lavender is antibacterial and high in antioxidants. It is also a pleasant flavouring agent and can be used in salads as garnish; in tea; to flavour milk; and to infuse white spirits like gin, vodka, white rum and white wine. I haven't cooked much with it as much as I have cooked with gulab, but have been using it along with or as a replacement for rosemary, to flavour meats and carbs like potato and cauliflower.

LAVENDER HONEY SYRUP

Ingredients:

3 cups water
7–8 springs of culinary lavender
4 tsp honey
¼ tsp grated ginger

Method:

1) Cover and simmer lavender and ginger in water in a pan for about 20–30 minutes.
2) Strain out the ginger and lavender and keep the water.

3) Warm the water and add honey to it. Keep stirring
and heating till the honey dissolves completely. Your
lavender syrup is now ready for use. You can use this
syrup for making lemonades and cocktails and even
to dress salads.

LAVENDER AND PISTACHIO KULFI

Ingredients:

4 tbsp lavender and honey syrup
10–12 pistachios crushed
1 cardamom crushed
½ tin Milkmaid
100 ml coconut milk
100 ml fresh cream
2 tsp grated coconut
10–12 culinary lavender springs
½ tsp lemon rind
1 tsp chia seeds

Method:

Warm the lemon rind in honey and then mix all the
ingredients together and pour it into kulfi moulds. Freeze it
for 2–3 hours and serve, with maybe a dollop of syrup.

LAVENDER AND ROSEMARY POTATOES

250 gm baby potatoes
1 onion finely chopped

1 tsp garlic paste
2 tsp olive oil
1 tsp butter
1 green chilli chopped
1 tsp culinary lavender
¼ tsp dried rosemary
Salt to taste

Method:

1) In a kadai, heat olive oil and butter till the butter gives off its aroma.
2) Add in garlic paste followed by the chopped onion.
3) Stir in the rest of the ingredients.
4) Serve with grilled fish/chicken and salad.

GEINDA

The bright orange and yellow marigold, known popularly as geinda, has a mild peppery flavour and can be used as a colouring substitute for saffron. It can also be used for garnishing meats. Steeped in warm water it can be used to treat sore throats and boost immunity. I have used it to make mulled wine, marmalade and baked curd. My brother-in-law, Rahul Bose, who works at a supercool company that designs beauty products among many other things, has a passion for rustling up beverages. He uses geinda flowers to make cold brew coffee infusions. My colleague Shruti Anand uses these blooms to flavour her special paranthas.

SPICY FLORAL MULLED WINE

It is a drink that has now become an integral part of my Christmas Eve party. Every year, I have an open house party on 24 December to ring in Christmas and my father's birthday. While the main dish and starters change, the plum cake and the mulled wine have always remained a constant.

Ingredients:

3 bottles of port wine
250 ml dark rum
4 oranges sliced into rounds
200 ml orange juice
2 cinnamon sticks
8 cloves
6 star anise
8–10 black peppercorns
1–2 tsp honey
4 dried hibiscus flowers
100 gm geinda flowers thoroughly washed and cleaned
Vanilla essence as per taste

Method:

1) Dry-roast all the spices and hibiscus flowers and stir it into the dark rum. This can be mixed and kept for 3–4 days prior or it can be left overnight.
2) In a large container pour the wine and let it simmer on low flame. I have started using a rice cooker to make it.

3) Add the spiced rum, honey, orange juice and vanilla essence and 'Cook' it in the rice cooker for about ten minutes.
4) Switch the cooker to 'Warm' mode and add in the orange slices. Stir it from time to time.
5) Serve it warm in wine glasses with a geinda floating on top—the flower has a strong flavour which seeps into the drink when served warm.

MARIGOLD AND ORANGE MARMALADE

Ingredients:

8–10 geinda flowers thoroughly washed and cleaned
3 oranges
3 tbsp sugar
1 tsp honey
5–6 cloves
1 lal mirch diced
½ tsp cornflour
2 cups water

Method:

1) Peel the oranges and extract the juice.
2) Clean the orange peels so that there's no thread or skin attached to it.
3) Cut the peels into small pieces.
4) Separate out the petals from the whole geinda flowers and keep them aside.

5) Warm the water and add in orange juice and sugar.

6) Once the sugar dissolves, add honey, cloves, geinda petals and lal mirch.

7) Simmer it all for 20–30 minutes.

8) Stir in cornflour and allow it to simmer till the mixture attains a jelly-like consistency.

9) Take it off the flame and allow it to cool down. Transfer it into a clean, dry glass jar and your marmalade is ready.

MARIGOLD AND SAFFRON BAKED CURD

Ingredients:

5–6 geinda flowers washed and cleaned
6–8 strands of saffron
1 can of Milkmaid
1 litre full-cream milk
1 tbsp milk powder
500 gm curd
2 tbsp grated cheese
2 tsp marigold and orange marmalade (optional)
25 gm nuts and dry fruits chopped

Method:

1) Transfer the curd on to a clean muslin cloth and hang it overnight or at least for four hours.

2) Heat the milk and, while it simmers, stir in milk powder.

3) When the powder dissolves in the milk, add geinda petals, saffron strands and grated cheese.

4) Let it all bubble and attain a golden-yellow hue.

5) Take it off the flame and mix in Milkmaid, hung curd and chopped nuts and dry fruits. You can mix the marmalade if you wish.

6) Transfer it into a baking dish and bake it at 100–120 degrees Celsius for sixty minutes.

7) Let it cool down and then keep it in the refrigerator for about two hours before serving.

COLD BREW COFFEE WITH MARIGOLD BY RAHUL BOSE

Ingredients:

30 ml cold brew coffee
30 ml coconut water
30 ml gin
1 geinda flower
Ice as needed

Method:

1) Chill a highball glass and put ice cubes in.

2) Pour the gin over the ice, followed by coconut water and cold brew coffee.

3) Float a geinda flower on top as garnish.

PARAT PARANTHA WITH MARIGOLD BY SHRUTI ANAND

Ingredients:

5 cups atta
Salt to taste
½ tsp *ajwain*/carom seeds
1 onion finely chopped
1 tsp coriander leaves finely chopped (optional)
Handful of geinda flower petals
Desi ghee

Method:

1) Mix atta, water, ghee and salt to knead into a soft dough.
2) Roll it out to make a square parantha; keep it a little thick. Layer the top of the parantha with desi ghee.
3) Sprinkle little ajwain, chopped onions, coriander leaves and geinda petals on it. Gently press these into the parantha.
4) Cut the parantha into diamond-shaped pieces with a knife.
5) Place layers one above the other and press it from the top to bind them together.
6) Then roll that out into a parantha.
7) Put it on the tawa with a bit of ghee.
8) Cook both sides and serve hot with spicy pickle or chutney.

APRAJITA

The blue peony or butterfly pea flower, what we know in India as the aprajita flower, is fast acquiring a cult status in gourmet food, especially in the world of beverages. This dainty flower is offered to Goddess Kali and it has a very calming effect. Chef Radhika Khandelwal has already shared a recipe with it. My own experimenting with this flower has yielded three recipes.

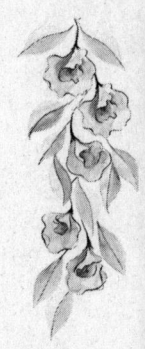

APRAJITA AND LAVENDER TEA

Ingredients for the blend:

500 gm white tea
100 gm culinary lavender
100 gm dried aprajita flowers
3–4 cardamoms crushed
2 tsp saunf/*mouri*

I mix them all together and keep it in an airtight container.

Method:

1) For a cup of tea, take one cup of water and bring it to a boil.
2) Lower the flame and add a teaspoon of the tea blend.

3) Switch off the flame, cover the vessel and let the tea brew for a minute.
4) Strain out the blue-hued tea in a transparent teacup.
5) Serve it with a wedge of lime on the side.

Watch the colour of the tea change when you put a drop of lime juice in it!

APRAJITA SANGRIA

Ingredients:

2 bottles of white wine
250 ml white rum or gin
1 bottle of sparkling wine
1 tbsp sugar
2 tsp honey
200 gm dried aprajita flowers
100 gm culinary lavender
1 tsp lavender extract
5–6 mint leaves crushed
2 apples diced

Method:

1) Mix all the ingredients together and let it mull for about 4–8 hours.
2) Serve in wine glasses with ice and an aprajita flower as garnish.

BLUE PEONY RICE

While hunting for recipes for the book I came across this indigo-coloured rice in my friend Geeta Rao's Instagram—@geetaslist. Geeta is the former beauty director of *Vogue*, India. Even as she is an authority on beauty she is fast becoming a sensitive food connoisseur. She shared with me the picture of a Thai rice dish which includes the blue peony or the aprajita flower. Based on the tastes and flavours that Geeta could remember, I set to work on the recipe and have achieved success in the same. Of course, my recipe it is not authentic Thai, rather it has a very Bengali touch to it.

Ingredients:

1 cup *gobindobhog* rice (a rice grain used in Bengali households to make *payesh*. It has a sticky texture and, therefore, my choice for this dish)
10–12 dried edible aprajita flowers chopped
2 tsp ginger finely chopped
3 cardamoms smashed
1 gondhorajlebu leaf
5–6 basil leaves chopped
2 ripe red chilli finely chopped
6–7 black peppercorns crushed
100 gm spring onion chopped
2 tbsp peanuts roasted and chopped
Salt to taste
Sugar to taste
2 tbsp refined oil

2 gondhorajlebu cut into small wedges
1 tsp sesame seeds

Method:

1) Soak the rice in water for 30–40 minutes.
2) Drain out the water and measure the rice after it has expanded.
3) Soak the aprajita flowers in a small cup of water to extract the colour and flavour. Strain out the water and keep it aside.
4) Make a paste with the flowers and keep it aside.
5) Heat oil in a kadai and add the ginger, cardamoms and black peppercorns.
6) Add the rice, flower water and flower paste and mix it all well.
7) Add salt, sugar and gondhorajlebu leaf. Cover and cook rice, adding water as necessary.
8) When the rice is cooked through, take it off the flame and transfer it to a serving bowl.
9) Fry garlic, basil leaves, chilli, peanuts, spring onions and sesame seeds and pour it over the rice. Serve with phoolkopi, chicken or prawn malai curry with a wedge of gondhorajlebu.

CALENDULA

Another humble flower that is making some noise in the culinary world is calendula. The flower has been used in beauty treatments for its gentle healing powers.

Calendula is often referred to as marigold and, therefore, it should not be confused with geinda, which is also called marigold.

BEETROOT, BLACK GRAPE AND CALENDULA SMOOTHIE BOWL BY GEETA RAO

According to Geeta, it is better to eat your smoothie than drink it, and this no-cereal smoothie bowl packs in an antioxidant punch. Calendula flowers are anti-inflammatory and soothing and they add a pretty touch of colour too.

Ingredients:

1 small beetroot (boiled)
6–10 black grapes (depending on size)
50 gm yogurt
6 chopped walnuts and almonds (three each)
2 tbsp finely chopped apple, pineapple and pear (crunchy fruits add a nice bite)
2–3 calendula flowers (petals only, thoroughly washed and cleaned)
1 tsp honey (optional)

Method:

1) Blend together beetroot, grapes and yogurt.
2) Pour into a bowl.
3) Top up with nuts, fruits, flowers and honey.

SOME OTHER BLOOMS

Apart from the five flowers mentioned above, here are some recipes with popular blossoms.

RAINBOW POHA BY GEETA RAO

Sweet and savoury, poha is a popular breakfast option across the country. This particular version of the humble dish is bright, colourful and flavourful. It has been created by Geeta, and here's what she has to say about it:

'I was inspired by the *phoolonwaalimehendi*, a lovely pre-wedding ritual where the bride is decked in fresh flowers instead of jewellery. So much more authentic! Poha is an easy-to-make breakfast and teatime snack, and this gives it a nice colourful twist and looks great when you are entertaining.

'When using edible flowers, ensure that they are from a known source, as they are so delicate you don't usually wash them. Discard stems of larger flowers and keep the very tender tiny stems of smaller flowers. You can chop larger flowers like nasturtiums, but be gentle. Use smaller flowers like viola and sweet william whole, as they are so pretty.'

Ingredients for cooking and tempering:

1 cup *jaada poha* (thick variety)
1 tsp black *rai* seeds
1 tsp cumin seeds
2 green chillies finely chopped

¼ cup fresh flowering coriander chopped fine
1 tsp lime juice
½ tsp powdered sugar (optional)
¼ cup roasted cashews and peanuts mixed

Ingredients for tossing and finishing:

½ cup freshly shredded coconut
3 large basil leaves torn or roughly chopped
1 tsp zest of lime (use a slightly thick-skinned fragrant lime)
2 tbsp of fresh turmeric grated to the same length as coconut
½ cup mixed edible flowers—calendula, viola, nasturtium, purple and green basil, and marigold. Set aside a couple of whole flowers for garnishing.

Method:

1) Wash poha well in a colander a couple of times; add salt to taste and mix well, and wait five minutes.
2) In a frying pan, heat a teaspoon of oil and let rai seeds and cumin seeds pop.
3) Add green chillies.
4) Add the poha and mix well.
5) Add sugar.
6) Add lime juice.
7) Mix again, shut lid and let it all integrate for a minute.
8) Switch off heat and rest for two minutes. Transfer on to the countertop.
9) Open lid and mix the contents of the coconut, zest of lime, basil and flower-infused bowl into the poha.

10) Mix well. Garnish with the saved whole flowers and
a handful of pomegranate seeds if handy.

This is best made and served fresh, as the flowers will not do
well with reheating. The recipe can be adapted to barley and
quinoa as well.

FLORAL TEA-TOX BY APARNA GUPTA

Aparna gravitates towards flowers whether they are blooming
in the garden, being sold by a vendor or as prints on clothes.
Her kitchen is also fragrant with the floral teas that she brews.
This tea blend, she says, 'is excellent to lift my spirits, as rose,
lavender and jasmine all are known for their ability to relieve
stress and anxiety. Being rich in antioxidants, they also help
to clear up the skin'.

Ingredients:

2 cups water freshly boiled
5–6 dried rose buds
1 tsp dried jasmine flowers
½ tsp lavender (it tends to get bitter)
½ tsp green tea (optional)
½ tsp honey (optional)

Method:

Place the ingredients in a small teapot. Add some hot water.
Steep for 2–3 minutes depending on the intensity of flavours
desired. This recipe makes two cups of tea.

MAHUA-INFUSED RUM BY PRIYADARSHINI GHOSH SAXENA

Priyadarshini is my cousin and an excellent cook. We are indeed a family of talented people. Here's a cool recipe of a flavoured rum from her kitchen.

Ingredients:

1 big cinnamon stick
4–5 star anise
½ tsp saunf
5–6 black peppercorns
3–4 cloves
2–4 drops mahua oil
750 ml dark rum

Method:

1) Dry-roast all the spices on a tawa.
2) When the spices start oozing their fragrance, take them off the flame.
3) Take a cup of dark rum, pour it into a saucepan and warm it a little.
4) Add to it the roasted spices and simmer it on low flame for a couple of minutes.
5) Pour it back into the bottle of rum and let it cool down.
6) Then add few drops of mahua oil and store it for 7–10 days.
7) Serve it the way you like having rum.

MILK OF PARADISE BY MEGHDOOT BOSE

This is a cocktail that my husband, Meghdoot, developed, drawing inspiration from Baileys Irish Cream. He is quite a good cook and an excellent mixologist.

Ingredients for making infusion:

750 ml vodka
2 drops of blue lotus essential oil
8–10 dried aprajita flowers

Method for making infusion:

1) Put the flowers and blue lotus oil in a bottle of vodka and let it rest for ten days.
2) Shake up the bottle every day to allow the ingredients to blend well.
3) Strain out the aprajita flowers. Use a filter paper to do it for best results.
4) Pour the now flavoured-vodka back into the bottle and store it.

Ingredients for cocktail:

30 ml flavoured vodka
2 tsp coconut milk
½ tsp honey
1–2 aprajita flowers
3–4 pieces of pineapple
Ice as much as you need

Method for cocktail:

1) Blend together vodka, coconut milk, honey and pineapple in a food processor.
2) Fill a highball glass with ice.
3) Pour the vodka blend over the ice.
4) Garnish with an aprajita flower and serve.

CONCLUSION:
TURNING POISON INTO MEDICINE

This book is my proof that a setback in life can become an opportunity. In my case it was my illness that pushed me not just to heal myself but also become a healer. I hope *Phoolproof* has encouraged you to transform your life and make you bloom to your true potential.

Having said that, my deepest desire is to have each one reading this book develop a relationship with flowers. Spend a little time each day with flowers—plant them, tend to them and watch them flourish. It would be a good idea to spend about twenty minutes meditating with flowers. Here's how you can start:

1) Take four drops of a flower essence in a glass of water.
2) Select a quiet and comfortable place to sit and meditate.
3) Choose a fresh bloom and hold it in your hand.
4) Inhale the fragrance of the flower and close your eyes.

5)   Take long deep breaths and observe your mind, body and breathing.

6)   When your breathing becomes slow and steady, start humming.

7)   Visualize yourself as a butterfly or bee in a gorgeous flower garden and continue humming.

8)   After about ten minutes, stop humming and just feel the energy washing through your body.

9)   Enjoy this moment of quiet and peace.

10) Slowly rub your palms together, inhale the flower again and gently open your eyes. Bless the Universe and accept the blessings of the Universe.

May each one of you bloom and grow, forever.

SUGGESTIONS FOR FURTHER READING

There is exhaustive literature on flowers. The more you read about them, the closer you will get to knowing flowers, and that's never a bad idea. To expand your repertoire of poems, folklores, fables and flowers, refer to the books mentioned below:

1. Amarjeet Singh Batth, *Home Gardener's Guide Indian Garden Flowers* (Bareilly, India: Prakash Book Depot, 2015).
2. Anna Jeoffroy and Philip Salmon, *Dr Bach's Flower Remedies: Tapping into the Positive Emotional Qualities of the Chakras including Annasation Technique* (Kindle Edition, 2013).
3. Stefan Ball, *The Batch Flower Remedies Workbook* (United Kingdom: The C.W. Daniel Company Ltd, 1998).
4. Beata Zatorska and Simon Target, *Rose Petal Jam: Recipes and Stories from a Summer in Poland* (n.p: Tabula Books, 2011).

5. Burton Watson, *The Lotus Sutra* (West Sussex: Columbia University Press, 1993).

6. Cathy Brown, *The Edible Flower Garden: From Garden to Kitchen: Choosing, Growing and Cooking Edible Flowers* (London: Southwater, 2014).

7. Chandler Burr, *The Emperor of Scent: A True Story of Perfume and Obsession* (New York: Random House Trade Paperbacks, 2004).

8. Christina Anthis, *There's Food on Your Face: The Hippie Homemaker's DIY Guide to Natural Health & Beauty* (North Carolina: Cary Press, 2014).

9. Cicely Mary Barker, *How to Host a Flower Fairy Tea Party* (Warne, 2004).

10. Cynthia Bourgeault, *The Meaning of Mary Magdalene: Discovering the Woman at the Heart of Christianity* (Boston: Shambhala, 2010).

11. Dan Burstein, *Secrets of Mary Magdalene* (Great Britain: Orion Publishing Group, 2007).

12. Dawn Cooper, *Shakespeare on Flowers: Panorama Pops* (United Kingdom: Walker Books Ltd, 2016).

13. Deborah Craydon and Warren Bellows. *Floral Acupuncture: Applying the Flower Essences of Dr Bach to Acupuncture Sites* (Crossing Press: 2015).

14. Dr Daisaku Ikeda, *Flowers of Hope* (New Delhi: Eternal Ganges Press Pvt. Ltd, 2013).

15. ———, *The Heart of the Lotus Sutra* (First Indian Edition, New Delhi: Eternal Ganges Press Pvt. Ltd, 2014).

16. Dr Edward Bach and F.J. Wheeler, *The Bach Flower Remedies* (New York: McGraw Hill Education, 1998).

17. Dr Edward Bach, *The Story of the Travellers and Other Remedy Stories* (United Kingdom: The Bach Centre, 2014).

18. ———, *Writings of Dr Edward Bach: Heal Thyself & the Twelve Healers and Other Remedies* (Kindle Edition, 2014).

19. Dr Malti Khaitan, *Flowers That Heal* (India: Atbs Publisher, 2010).

20. Dr Rachel Herz, *The Scent of Desire: Discovering Our Enigmatic Sense of Smell* (New York: William Morrow, 2007).

21. Dr Ravi Ratan, *Handbook of Aromatherapy: A Complete Guide to Essential & Carrier Oils, Their Application & Therapeutic Use for Holistic Health & Wellbeing* (Delhi: Motilal Banarsidass, 2009).

22. Dr V. Krishnamoorty, *Beginner's Guide to Bach Flower Remedies* (India: B. Jain Large Print, 2009).

23. Elisabeth Barille, *Guerlain* (New York: Assouline Publishing, 2011).

24. *Essential Oils for Beginners: The Guide to Get Started with Essential Oils and Aromatherapy* (United States: Althea Press, 2013).

25. Gill Farrer-Halls, *The Aromatherapy Bible: The Definitive Guide to Using Essential Oils* (London: Gods Field Press, 2005).

26. Hayley Anderson, *Faith Flower* (Kindle Edition, 2016).

27. Holger Kersten, *Jesus Lived in India* (New Delhi: Penguin Books India Pvt. Ltd, 1986).

28. Ian White, *Australian Bush Flower Healing* (Australia: Random House, 1999).

29. Indu Sunderesan, *The Feast of Roses: A Novel* (New York: Washington Square Press, 2004).

30. Isabel Bercaw and Caroline Bercaw, *Bath Bombs, Body Scrubs & More! Over 50 Natural Bath And Beauty Recipes for Beautiful Skin* (n.p: Crestline Books, 2019).

31. Jane Holloway. *The Language of Flowers: Poem* (London: Everyman's Library, 2017).

32. Jessica Ress, *100 Organic Skin Care Recipes* (United States: Adams Media, 2014).

33. Jill Winch, *Painting Flowers* (London: Arcturus Publishing Ltd, 2001).

34. Jo Malone, *Jo Malone: My Story* (London: Simon & Schuster, 2016).

35. John Herlihy, *Somewhere a Flower Blooms: Poems on the Human Condition* (Florida: Ansar Books, 2016).

36. Judy Ramsell Howard, *Bach Flower Remedies for Women* (London: C.W. Daniel, 1992).

37. Judy Ramsell Howard, *The Bach Flower Remedies Step by Step: A Complete Guide to Selecting and Using the Remedies* (United Kingdom: Vermillion, 2005).

38. Julie Gabriel, *Green Beauty Recipes* (United Kingdom: CreateSpace Independent Publishing Platform, 2013).

39. Juliette Goggin and Abi Righton, *Handmade Beauty: Natural Recipes for Your Face, Body and Hair* (London: Jacqui Small, 2016).

40. Karen Gilbert, *Natural Beauty: 35 Step-by-step Projects for Homemade Beauty* (Kindle Edition; CICO Books; Reprint Edition, 2015).

41. Lisa Reddings. *Organic Perfume: The Complete Beginners Guide & 50 Best Recipes for Making Heavenly, Non-Toxic Organic DIY Perfumes from Your Home! (Aromatherapy, Essential Oils, Homemade Perfume)* (California: CreateSpace Independent Publishing Platform, 2015).

42. Margaret Roberts, *100 Edible & Healing Flowers: Cultivating, Cooking, Restoring Health* (South Africa: Penguin Random House, 2014).

43. Margaret Starbird, *The Woman with the Alabaster Jar: Mary Magdalen and the Holy Grail* (Rochester: Bear & Company, 1993).

44. Mechthild Scheffer. *The Encyclopedia of Bach Flower Therapy* (Healing Arts Press, 2001).

45. Meena Arora Nayak, *The Blue Lotus: Myths and Folktales of India* (New Delhi: Aleph Book Company, 2018).

46. Michael Baigent, Richard Leigh and Henry Lincoln, *Holy Blood, Holy Grail: The Secret History of Christ. The Shocking Legacy of the Grail* (New York: Dell, 2015).

47. Miche Bacher, *Cooking with Flowers: Sweet and Savory Recipes with Rose Petals, Lilacs, Lavender, and Other Edible Flowers* (Philadelphia: Quirk Books, 2013).

48. Mireille Guiliano, *French Women for All Seasons: A Year of Secrets, Recipes, & Pleasure* (United States: Vintage Books, 2009).

49. Nikos Kazantzakis, *The Last Temptation* (New York: Simon & Schuster, 1998).

50. Nimret Handa, *Wild Flowers of India* (New Delhi: Full Circle Publishing, 2018).

51. Rebecca Sullivan, *The Art of Edible Flowers: Recipes and Ideas for Floral Salads, Drinks, Desserts And More* (United Kingdom: Kyle Books, 2018).

52. Rosalind Creasy, *The Edible Flower Garden* (Singapore: Periplus Edition, 1999).

53. Rupi Kaur, *The Sun and Her Flowers* (Kansas City, Missouri: Andrews McMeel Publishing, 2017).

54. Sahara Rose Ketabi, *Eat Feel Fresh: A Contemporary, Plant-based Ayurvedic Cookbook* (n.p: Alpha, 2018).

55. Sally White, *Essential Oils and Flowers: Healing Your Mind, Body and Spirit* (California: Create Space Independent Pub, 2015).

56. Stacey Dugliss-Wesselman and Susan Gregg, *Herbal Remedies Made Simple: A Beginner's Guide to Using Plants, Herbs, and Flowers for Health and Well-Being* (n.p: Fair Winds Press, 2018).

57. Star Khechara, *The Holistic Beauty Book* (United Kingdom: Totnes, 2008).

58. Stephen Buchmann, *The Reason for Flowers: Their History, Culture and Biology* (New York: Scribner, 2015).

59. Suparna Trikha, *The Book of Natural Skincare* (Delhi: HarperCollins India, 1999).

60. Susan Curtis, *Neal's Yard Remedies Beauty Book* (Great Britain: DK, 2015).

61. Susan Goldman Ruben, *Coco Chanel: Pearls, Perfume, and the Little Black Dress* (New York: AbRams The Art of Books, 2018).

62. Tilar J. Mazzeo, *The Secret of Chanel No. 5: The Intimate History of the World's Most Famous Fragrance* (n.p: Harper Perennial, 2011).

63. Valerie Ann Worwood, *The Complete Book of Essential Oils and Aromatherapy: Over 800 Natural, Nontoxic, and Fragrant Recipes to Create Health, Beauty, and Safe Home and Work Environments* (United States: New World Library, 2016).

64. Vanessa Diffenbaugh, *The Language of Flowers: A Novel* (United States: Ballentine Books, 2011).

AFTERWORD

It's been just over ten years since I met Jhelum Biswas Bose, when she was the beauty editor of *Harper's Bazaar India*. She was always the first to arrive at the office, and almost the favourite part of my day would be our morning catch-up. She was always positive, authentic and had a daily beauty tip for me: the nail polish that was the most chip-resistant, the face oil that would add that natural glow to my skin . . .

Beauty was in her blood; her mom worked in the industry and positivity and radiance are just a part of her aura. Natural beauty was an obvious path for her (and she studied alternative healing therapy), but of course she has found her own beautiful connection—to flowers!

Jhelum, through this book, has taught me how to embrace my own inner flower child. There is nothing that gives more pleasure than arranging fresh flowers in vases all around my house. And when I am feeling down, I often use them as a focal point for some deep thinking. Thanks to Jhelum, I know now how flowers are therapeutic in so many ways and the science behind them.

I have already started adding crab apple essence to my face cream and will be stocking up on my jasmine oil on my next trip to India. And I can't wait to try the aprajita and lavender tea recipe she suggests.

Everyone who has an affinity to flowers will relate to this book—and it is bound to bring some cheer to your life.

Sujata Assomull
Founding editor, *Harper's Bazaar India*

ACKNOWLEDGEMENTS

Accomplishing any endeavour always requires team effort. Even the solitary job of a writer needs inspiration, help, reference, experience, encouragement, pampering, critiquing and, most importantly, the belief and faith of the people in her life, to pull off a book. I feel truly blessed to have many such persons in my life, starting with my parents—Ruby and Arjun Biswas. It is my mother's fierce encouragement and my father's silent but rock-solid support that have been my driving force. Much like my father, my husband, Meghdoot, has been a quiet yet steady strength. I can't thank him enough for bearing with my eccentric experiments that engulfed (I believe enveloped) our home, starting with my study; then the kitchen, the place of execution; and finally the table and our living spaces and social discussions.

My heartfelt gratitude to my sister, Arpita; my cousins Satyajit and Prosenjit; my sisters-in-law Nandini, Meghna, Shradhha and Shipra; my brothers-in-law, Joydeb and Rahul; and my friends Alpana, Rhythma, Swati, Deepa, Dona, Varun, Sutapa, Amit, Moonmoon and Kshama for being kind enough to read my writing and sharing their valuable feedback. A special thanks to my colleague and confidante Shruti for painstakingly going through the manuscript and being a calming presence in my crazy life. Many thanks to Sarang for carving out time from his super-busy schedule to click my 'author photos'.

I am grateful to my parents-in-law, Chandra and Aloke Bose, for their encouragement, blessings and the pride they take in my achievements.

Many thanks to my sounding board, source of solace and reservoir of compassionate encouragement, Joyshri Sen, without whom I would be lost in some dark tunnel.

I am grateful to all those who generously contributed to the book with their secret recipes, experiments and reviews. Lisa, thank you for so kindly writing the foreword to this book; and Sujata, many thanks for writing the afterword and, as always, guiding me through all my career moves.

Gurveen, thank you for believing I could write this book and being such an excellent editor. Joseph, you have shaped my copy into a sharp, crisp read—my deep gratitude to you.

My deepest respect for my teachers—GJV Prasad, Saugata Bhaduri and Bertram Da Silva—who honed my writing skills, and to late Anna Jeoffroy who taught me the basics of Bach flower remedy.

Radhika, Debarpann, Coco and Ahaan—my nieces and nephews—I hope through this book I was able to inspire you to chase your dreams in life.

However, nothing would have been the way it has been had it not been for my eternal mentor Dr Daisaku Ikeda, whose regular messages gave me the strength to write this book of flowers, colours, tastes, sensations, myths, healing and poetry, when I was going through the darkest phase of my life. The lotus indeed blooms in the muddy pond; misery can be the fuel for creativity.

A NOTE ON THE AUTHOR

Born and brought up in Kolkata, Jhelum Biswas Bose developed her aesthetics early on, with her mother in the beauty business and father in photography. Her city made her a bibliophile, and later she pursued a master's and an MPhil in English literature in Jawaharlal Nehru University. A lover of Keats's poetry, she did not want to change from an incorrigible Romantic into a critic, which is what the academic profession requires. So she decided to tap into her heritage and join the India Today Group, and work as a beauty editor for a decade for lifestyle magazines such as *Harper's Bazaar*, *Good Housekeeping* and *Women's Health*. Thereafter, she took up the role of marketing head for Sephora India.

In 2014, Jhelum had to take a sabbatical from work due to ill health. However, this proved to be a boon: Her Buddhist practice gave her the tools to self-reflect, focus and understand how she could serve others. As she healed herself with alternative therapies, she began learning them as well. She started a website on beauty—www.beautybeats.in—and created a collection of beauty products called Jhelum Loves.

Jhelum is trained in Bach flower remedies and aromatherapy, and has developed her own way of healing, called 'Phoolproof Therapy'. She also contributes to various lifestyle magazines and writes poems and short stories. In 2019 she moved to Bengaluru and now divides her time between three cities—Kolkata, Delhi and Bengaluru—surrounded by fairies, flowers, friends, family and some animals.